High Praise for *"Shut Up, Skinny Bitches!"*

"Stop dieting, and start living—today. This book will show you how! And I guarantee you will laugh along the way."

—Jenni Schaefer
Author of *"Life Without Ed: How One Woman Declared Independence from Her Eating Disorder and How You Can Too"* and *"Goodbye Ed, Hello Me: Recover from Your Eating Disorder and Fall in Love with Life"*

"The authors artfully combine compassion, confrontation, and common sense as they dispel the myths that drive so many people into eating disorders. In their honest and open dialogues, they connect readers not only to the facts, but also to the motivation to change—a refreshing approach. This book is a must-read for anyone who's been tempted to engage in disordered eating, for those who are experiencing an eating disorder, and for those who care about them and want to help."

—Pat Santucci, MD, FAPA, FAED,
Executive Vice President, National Association
of Anorexia Nervosa and Associated Disorders (ANAD)

"Rago and Archer in *Shut Up, Skinny Bitches!* eloquently look at the need to empower oneself in the fight against unhealthy dieting. They have looked at the myths and truths in the dieting culture. This book will help readers become free from the overpowering/influential diet culture."

—Steven M. Prinz, M.D.,
Author of *The Anxious Brain*

"An excellent common sense book that gets right to the heart of the matter of why so many of us suffer from body-image crisis. *Shut Up, Skinny Bitches!* gives readers the assurance that forcing ourselves to be unnaturally thin is not the answer to anyone's self-esteem problems. Rago and Archer expose the mindset that you're only worthwhile if you're a double-size zero. They show that in the case of loving yourself, size truly doesn't matter... This is a must-read!"

—Kristen Houghton
Author of *And Then I'll Be Happy*

Shut Up, Skinny Bitches!

The Common Sense Guide to Following Your Hunger and Your Heart

Maria Rago PhD & Greg Archer

Printed in the United States of America

ISBN: 978-1-935254-32-4

Cover Inspiration by Joshua Becker
Illustrations by Vanda Grigorovic
Book Design by Nadene Carter

First printing, 2011

Dedication

If you've ever starved yourself or felt ashamed of your body – this book is dedicated to you. We wish you healing, love, and peace.

To Alex and Tia Khan – creative, supportive, knowledgeable, and concerned for our world. You could never fully know my love and admiration for you.   —Mom

To Cousin Chris, who never stopped believing in me, and to the close friends who've listened – a lot! – and whose love continues to inspire me to be a better human being.   —Greg

Totus tuus.

Dedication

If you've ever starved yourself or felt ashamed of your body – this book is dedicated to you. We wish you healing, love, and peace.

To Alex and Tia Khan – creative, supportive, knowledgeable, and concerned for our world. You could never fully know my love and admiration for you.   —Mom

To Cousin Chris, who never stopped believing in me, and to the close friends who've listened – a lot! – and whose love continues to inspire me to be a better human being.   —Greg

Totus tuus.

Table of Contents

Introduction

ARE YOU SICK AND TIRED OF SKINNY BITCHES saying you're too fat, you don't fit in, and you'll never be good enough? We are. After sifting through a smorgasbord of so-called diet and health books during our lifetime, we still find it hard to believe the underlying messages in most of these books are exactly the same: everyone needs to be thinner; losing weight cures self-hatred; and people are fat because, basically, they're stupid.

The nerve!

Well, we know you're hungry for something delicious to sink your teeth into. So, put down the diet soda and pick up a cupcake. We're here to tell you the messages in most diet and health books feed into the self-destructive, fear-based attitudes prevalent in America and beyond. And they hardly deliver their promised result: that you'll be thin, and when you are, your life will be fabulous. We offer a smart, alternative, common sense guide to following your hunger and your heart when it comes to eating well and feeling good about yourself. And you'll find this has little to do with being thin.

over the years, that freaky diet-book orgy somehow
~~~ we like to call a Skinny Bitches Mindset (SBM).
It might be occupying a psyche near you. A SBM
...urotic anxiety with a major scoop of "you're not thin
enough because you don't eat correctly" tossed in for good measure.
This restrictive way of thinking creates a scenario with no room for
acceptance of who you are – no matter what size you wear. When
acceptance does arrive, it's reserved for the thinnest among us –
the elite. Everyone else is ... well ... a loser. Thus, the SBM excludes
people based on size, and it condones the notion that thin people
have more value than heavier ones. This judgmental attitude fuels
lack of self-esteem and acceptance of yourself and others.

Hard to digest? Hell, yes!

But make no mistake: we're not singling out the book *Skinny
Bitch*, the popular bestseller that quipped, "Stop being a moron and
start getting skinny." That book is just one of many bestsellers that
convey messages we disagree with, and it finally forced us to stand tall
and consider an alternative way of thinking about our relationship
with ourselves, our bodies, and food. Our book doesn't serve as an
overall commentary on *Skinny Bitch* the book; we're addressing
skinny bitches at-large, those in our culture who live and breathe the
SBM.[1] We're talking back to anyone who ever suggested we're not
good enough and anyone who *dares* suggest you're not good enough.

Listen up: the time has come to stop thinking you have to strut
your skinny ass down the street and prance around in a thong like
you rule the planet. You rule the world anyway, whether you're thin
or not. It's time to love your ass, no matter what shape it is. Time to
love the asses of your sisters and brothers out there, too. You're a
lovable person, and that has nothing whatsoever to do with the size
of your ass. You can feel good about what you're eating. But first, take
hold of any foul-mouthed critics, duct tape their pie holes, and join
us by shouting

Shut Up, Skinny Bitches!

---

[1] Though this book is not about *Skinny Bitch*, we do have strong opinions about the
book's superior tone. Read our thoughts in a book review found in the epilogue.

*"I'm awfully sorry for people who are
taken in by all of today's dietary mumbo jumbo.
They are not getting any enjoyment out of their food."*
—Julia Child

Chapter One
Shut Up, and Eat!

EAT! SKINNY IS NOT THE CURE. Neither is being a skinny bitch. So let's stop a moment and ponder a few things. If, like so many other folks out there who are trying to lose weight, you believe the sun will suddenly rise and shine brightly over the horizon of your skinny ass – once you *make* it skinny – and everything will just be divine when you're thin, you're bloated with a ton of misinformation. We'll say it again: skinny is *not* the cure.

A diet is. But not the kind you're thinking. The one we're proposing doesn't restrict eating. It doesn't force you to go to the gym seven times a week. It won't even make you work up a sweat – at least not physically. The only diet any of us need to go on is *The Inner Critic Fast*. You know what we're talking about. We're all so intimate with our inner crank, aren't we? And depending on where the mood is swinging, that inner critic can tell us any number of things: We're not good enough, we'll never amount to anything, or worse, we're overweight and don't look hot. Ever!

Don't you get enough criticism from people around you? We thought so. We really don't need any more, especially when it comes from inside ourselves.

We can thumb through all the psych books, cull from our own inner growth and professional experience, and come up with a brainiac answer for you, but we know you may be too busy obsessing about being skinny – we forgive you, by the way – so let's just slice some cheese and nibble away at this, shall we?

We've come to believe our inner critics might be more alert and out of control these days because we're all more susceptible than ever before to the messages in society and the media. This is the 21st century after all. And with all the Tweeting, Facebooking, and celeb-obsessing we all seem to do, hasn't it become more challenging to disengage from those subconscious messages we're being fed? Those messages include...

Skinny people are better than fat people.
Skinny people are more popular.
Skinny people are more successful.
Skinny people have better relationships.
Skinny people are happier.
Skinny people are perfect.

Welcome to the Skinny Bitches Mindset found in numerous diet and health books. The SBM has ballooned over the last twenty years and continues its revolutionary expansion. The message is clear: to be happy or successful, you must first be thin.

Wrong!

What's so important about being thin? Usually, health reasons are cited, but many people at a healthy weight still crave being thinner. Thin. Thin. Thin. Yawn!

We've learned an overweight person can improve his or her health by losing only a small amount of weight. Furthermore, underweight people can vastly improve their health by gaining weight. These facts are ignored in our thin-obsessed world. Even the medical community is affected by the SBM.

Still, our culture's thinness worship goes way beyond the guise of health. Just take a look at those magazines at the grocery store checkout line. (We know you do.) If some celeb du jour like Angelina Jolie gains a pound, the media eats it up. (Ever wonder what the media is really hungry for? Your attention, honey – and the coins in your pocket.) The thing is, the more people worship thinness, the more they subconsciously value restraining food intake. If you want to be thinner, you have to eat less, right? The two go hand in hand, like a knife and fork.

But what's so valuable about restricting food intake? What does this action say about you? Does it somehow make you a better person; someone who's in control? (Maybe to SBMers but not to us.) Why do people have to be blamed and shamed when they overeat, binge-eat, or simply eat normally?

We're here to set the record straight. Ample research indicates binge-eating is typically caused by restricting food or dieting. When people restrict food, they usually become so hungry they eat things they don't even want, until they simply can't stop. In fact, numerous studies illustrate that dieting *predicts* weight gain. (In research terms, prediction means *causes*.) Get it? The well-intentioned, compliant society member – that would be you – wishes to be accepted and loved, so she/he tries to please by restricting food. And how are you rewarded for your suffering? You binge-eat because you're hungry, and then YOU GAIN WEIGHT. Now, there's the rub.

And what's this? You also get to experience the shame and emotional pain of overeating, which is almost a cardinal sin. Excellent – now you'll never be good enough. You'll *never* be good like those skinny bitches. But you'll try again tomorrow. You say, "Yes, I'm a loser today, but I'll do better tomorrow." Guess what? You've bought into society's values so well that you can't even hear your own voice any more. That bitchy inner critic living inside the SBM is the only voice you hear.

Hello – where are you? Where's your voice? WAKE UP! Listen to it.

Your inner voice is trying to scream, "I'm hungry!" But the inner critic on the SBM network says, "That's why you're a loser. If you eat, you'll gain weight. If you gain weight, you're not acceptable, stupid!"

True or False? If you're overweight, you just need to stop eating so much. If you consumed less fat, fewer carbs, and fewer calories, you'd finally be healthy, thin, and fit in.

False! Surprise. Study after study reveals this belief is not true. Yet it seems like common sense, right? Eat less, lose weight, be beautiful, everything's fine.

Changing people's minds about this belief isn't easy. That's why it's imperative you listen to your own voice. Begin by repeatedly telling yourself you're strong enough to hop off this mental merry-go-round. Consider for a moment how much valuable time you waste by focusing on, "Oh, no, my stomach is too big. I'm fat!"

Ah, but you're not alone. Many of us experience this. Over the years, we've heard dozens of stories from people who struggle with these issues – Maria from her eating disorder patients; Greg from the many fitness students he has instructed.

Diane, a fifty-three-year-old nurse and proud grandmother recovering from an eating disorder, believed – as many of us often do – that she had to be thinner to fit in or be loved. She candidly shares with us...

> ❝I was always aware of body image and fatness, and I always knew that being fat, stout, pudgy, roly-poly, and such were bad things. I heard "skinny and cute" in my preschool years and knew that didn't apply to me. I remember baby fat being mentioned. My father always told me I was chubby from the

youngest age. But my dad wasn't fed much at home in his childhood, so any type of cooking was a treat to him, and he ate heartily whenever I dined with him. But in every breath between bites he told me and my sister how fat we were - or chubby - and that I ate too many pies and cookies. He truly never let up. Not a single stranger, mostly women, could pass by without a comment regarding weight, size, ugliness, or beauty. I lived with this throughout my adolescence, like the oxygen I breathed. But it was carbon monoxide to my psyche. 99

Dieting doesn't work, but this fact doesn't matter to most people. We keep trying again and again because we've lost control over our own decision-making. The culture tells us, "It's not the diet that's wrong, it's your hunger – you just shouldn't be so hungry." Do you see the white elephant standing in the living room of this insanity? The true message is, "Hunger is for losers." The implication is that if you just try harder, you'll finally succeed. People spend a lifetime battling hunger – and losing. Worse, they're always made to feel like terrible failures.

Can you relate? Are you caught up in an endless cycle of trying to restrict food and then beating yourself up as if every decision you make is wrong? Have you lost yourself because you're ruled by the SBM?

This question is key. How much time each day do you spend thinking about eating and your body image? Go ahead – think about it. Consider how that brainpower could be better used. If we all used every bit of our energy to be thin, how would we ever accomplish world peace? And there's so much more beyond war. We have energy issues to deal with and oil spills to clean up. Not to mention, millions of people on the planet don't even have enough food. Yet we're programmed to drain all our energy making sure our damn thighs don't touch.

Here's the thing: when you don't eat, you become pale, sunken, hungry, and ... well ... downright bitchy. People starve themselves so the skinny bitches of the world will accept them. Why are we so willing to conform, no matter what the cost?

Get this: being skinny does not cure self-hatred. (Skinny is not the cure, remember?) Actually, you can starve to death and be quite bitchy before you die. You'd get bitchier with each passing day. You would probably die from dehydration before starvation, which is how it happens. Yes, you can be a skinny dead bitch before you know it.

How do you stop bitching and start eating? Everything in moderation, baby. Yeah, it's that simple. (And we thank Ben Franklin for coining the phrase.) Begin to notice your thought patterns. (Yikes, right?) Relax. Just notice when that inner critic is making a mad dash toward a bunch of lies. (Remember lies sound like this: "I'm not good enough!" "I'm fat and ugly!" I'm worthless!" "There's something wrong with me!" "I can never change!")

Noticing these things will give you a sense of detachment – hopefully loving detachment. The very act of noticing creates the possibility for something else, some other thought or truth, to make itself known. Noticing your thoughts gives you an opportunity to make a choice. Think of it as a fork in the road (or the cheesecake). Noticing *what* you're thinking and simply questioning its validity will help you stop obsessing over every detail of what you're eating. You can begin to get in touch with your body again, because – and here's the great news – you were born knowing when you're hungry and when you're full. You don't need to hear about it from skinny bitches. You don't need to dwell on it. You simply need to be reminded of your spectacular nature. You need to remember what foods you liked before you started dieting, over-thinking, and picking apart every aspect of your body and eating regime.

One of the best things you can do: don't adhere to a list of *good* foods and *bad* foods. Make your own damn list and write down the foods you enjoy. But take note, eat those foods in moderation. Eat when you're hungry. Stop when you're full. (Boy, is it that simple? Yep.) It might be cool to add physical activity to the mix. Stir all this together and you may not be a skinny bitch, but you might actually enjoy your day for once. And, if the outcome is that you're thinner, good for you. But remember, skinny is not the cure.

Shut Up, About Being Skinny!

You were born knowing when you're hungry and when you're full. You don't need to be chastised about it by skinny bitches.

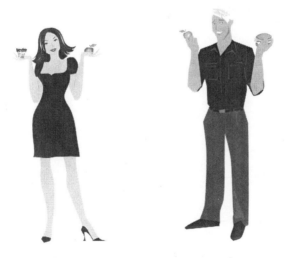

"Insanity is doing the same thing over and over again and expecting different results."

—Albert Einstein

Chapter Two
Epic Fail: Dieting

Dieting? We have three words for you. *Get over it.*

"But there's no other way for me to lose the weight I want to lose if I don't restrict some of my eating," you say. Or, "Gosh, my cousin's wedding is coming up, she's forcing me to wear that tight crimson gown for the bridal party, and if I don't drop, like, fifteen pounds real quick, then honey – I'm gonna look like one big fat tomato!"

Three more words. *Diets don't work.*

Here's the funny part. You already know this. In fact, we all know diets aren't effective. Not for the long haul, anyway. You might see temporary weight loss results, but inevitably, almost every dieter gains back the weight they lose, sometimes more. (Oprah, Kirstie, care to chime in?) In fact, in 2007 *American Psychologist* reported that an analysis of thirty-one studies of weight loss showed dieters initially lost 5 to 10 percent of their starting weight. But two years later, at least 83 percent gained back *more* weight than they originally lost. They would have been better off had they not dieted at all.

Have you noticed chronic dieters, and otherwise erratic or

restrictive eaters, are some of the most frustrated, depressed people you meet? They're always fighting themselves and their body's natural cravings. The emotional war with their bodies drains them of precious life energy. They seem forever lost and unhappy.

Are you a chronic dieter? No way! Everyone knows diets fail, right? You're just making a "lifestyle change," – the new lingo people use when they talk about dieting. The problem with that kind of lifestyle change is that it comes with a built-in implication: you're never supposed to get off your damn diet.

Trust us, the more rigid, restrictive, and guilt-ridden your "lifestyle change," the more it's a DIET. If you can relate to any of the following statements, you could be a chronic dieter.

1. I constantly worry about what I've eaten, am eating, or will eat.
2. I try to always make low-fat, low-carb, low-calorie choices.
3. I beat myself up when I don't make low-fat, low-carb, low-calorie choices.
4. Eating certain snacks, sweets, or foods makes me nervous. I make sure to make up for it later by restricting my food or exercising.

If you answered yes to any of the above statements, then good for you. You're honest. But listen to us: this book promotes eating. Healthy eating. (And yes, sometimes eating a cookie is the healthy thing to do.) The sooner we can all truly embrace the idea that it's okay to eat and actually eat regularly, then we can experience more peace and harmony in our lives. But don't freak out! We understand there's resistance to the idea of eating regularly. After all, nearly everywhere we look today, we find messages insisting there's something bad about food; that we should restrict our food consumption in some fashion and, of course, embark on any number of dieting escapades.

Just-juice diet, anyone? How about that grapefruit and watermelon diet? High-protein? Low-carbs?

How long has anyone lasted on any of these "miracle" weight loss plans or trendy "lifestyle changes?"

Don't diet. Eat!

We don't encourage you to make a glutton of yourself. We like you. We wouldn't do that. Don't be foolish. We don't condone eating entire gallons of Baskin Robbins ice cream every day or a box of donuts three times a week. We're simply pointing out that many foods, including snacks, taste so damn good that they're soothing for the soul. Shut up and consume some of these foods. It's okay. We promise.

Kim, a forty-six-year-old comic, playwright, mother, and wife living in Northern California, tells us...

> "I've been aware of my looks and my body from a very young age, not because I was blessed with "all that," but because I took hours of dance class from age five up, where I spent every afternoon in front of full-length mirrors. Add to that my involvement in theater, and I brewed the perfect concoction of vanity and self-doubt, constantly comparing myself and my physical appearance to other girls and women, usually falling short, yet forcing myself to try and fit an unattainable mold.
>
> Like many women, I was a successful yo-yo dieter in my twenties, losing and gaining enormous amounts of weight according to my social or performing schedule. In my thirties I had kids. Lots of them. In my forties I convinced myself to reclaim some athletic sense of myself and became deeply involved in an active, full-contact sport. My body built muscle, stamina, and endurance, but remained a size I didn't recognize as the ideal from childhood. My scale was steadily reading 200 pounds, which at 5'8" and by Hollywood standards was interplanetary in my twisted mind.

I visited a pair of professional trainers to assess my situation and horsewhip me into a shape I had preconceived notions of becoming. After an hour and a half of weighing, measuring, testing, and whatnot, their final evaluation of my fitness and goals threw me for an emotional loop that took days to grasp. My ideal weight is 170-180 pounds. I've never heard any woman utter this sentence, so I had to examine the facts. I am 46. I am sporadically athletic. I am strong. I am healthy. I am just about okay, and can choose to keep or lose twenty pounds. I can relax for the first time in my life and embrace the size 14. **"**

THE HEALTH POLICE

Let's face it, skinny bitches sit in their popularity castles and try to rule the world by sticking their bony derrieres out for all mankind to see. And the more we're flooded with those images, plus messages from mass media suggesting we simply must be thin to thrive in life, the more we believe we want what those skinny bitches are feeding us.

Maybe you had a little fight left in you. You know, to fend off the rejection and humiliation from the Skinny Bitches Mindset (SBM). Perhaps you were just about to conjure up the courage to say, "I *am* beautiful for who I am. I don't have to hate myself or others just because we don't measure up to a certain standard of beauty." But then the Health Police arrived, telling you, "Those skinny bitches are right! You aren't acceptable the way you are. You *are* too fat! And it's all because you don't eat correctly! AND BY THE WAY – YOU'RE GONNA DIE!"

Oh, the health police love to make us feel guilty about enjoying a nice snack. "Miss, put down the Cheetos and slowly step away from the kitchen counter." Good Lord! If you're found eating potato chips or cheesecake, an army of skinny bitches – plus a legion of parents, doctors, neighbors, gym teachers, politicians, and news reporters –

move in for the kill. They're quick to point out you're breaking some kind of law if you dare enjoy "unhealthy" food. Their main argument? Eating low-fat and low-calorie foods is always the best way to go. But is it?

No.

Research indicates that following a low-fat diet does *not* necessarily improve your health nor does it automatically create weight loss. Few know about this because most people believe low-fat *always* improves our health. Research to the contrary is ignored.

In 2006 a study of more than 48,000 women conducted by The Women's Health Initiative found that following a low-fat diet did *not* decrease the risk of heart attack, stroke, colon cancer, or breast cancer. Despite research showing that low-fat eating is an epic failure, the health police never bothered to share that information. In fact, David Kritchevsky, former professor of Philadelphia's Wistar Institute and an enigmatic contributor to the nation's debate on nutrition and health for nearly sixty years before his death in 2006, once noted that, **"In America, we no longer fear God, or the communists, but we fear fat."**

How true that is.

Revered journalist and author, Gary Taubes, wrote the 2007 page-turner *Good Calories, Bad Calories: Challenging the Conventional Wisdom on Diet, Weight Control, and Disease.* In a 2001 article in the journal *Science*, he wrote that political, social, and cultural processes actually shaped our intense fear of fat—not science. Science, he noted, hasn't determined if reduced dietary intake of fat improves our health. In fact, limiting fat may even be detrimental to our health.

Hello! Your beautifully robust brain is 60 percent fat, mostly to insulate your neurons. Severely changing fat consumption could impact membrane permeability in all the cells of your body, potentially impacting cellular processing of bacteria and viruses, plus all other cellular functions. Talk about mind-bending.

The possible negative effects of severely decreased dietary fat intake have not been studied. (What? No funding?) There's more interest, it seems, in health studies with one primary agenda – to prove eating fat is downright bad for us. (Which by the way, has never been proven.) Today, millions of people kick their own asses to eliminate fat from their diets. Worse, children are tortured about the foods they eat. Imagine a first-grader reading food labels. Why are third graders saying, "My teacher says we aren't allowed to eat that snack because it's unhealthy."

Sounds like adolescent boot camp for obsessive behavior.

There's no evidence that children *must* limit their dietary fat intake to be healthy. Couldn't this actually be unhealthy for them? Growing children may need fat intake even more than adults, and we don't understand the possible consequences of restricting fats and calories in children. Children require fat and calories so their bodies can grow in healthy ways. And don't fool yourself – they also need some fat intake for their *emotional* health. The health police and other skinny bitches come down hard on these kids, leaving them with the negative message: Something's wrong with them because they enjoy the food they love and crave. These messages are ingrained at an early age. No wonder we all have so many issues with food. We've even met adults who've never tasted a banana split because it's bad for them.

Pass them the hot fudge – *pronto*!

The participants cited earlier in the Women's Health Initiative study – the one indicating eating low-fat failed to provide any health benefit – pushed themselves to consume only 20 percent of their calories from fat. Through the first year of the study, the lower fat eaters weighed about five pounds less than the others. But after seven years of this "near draconian" regime – we're talking about women who constantly pushed themselves to restrict fat intake – the difference between women who avoided fat and ladies who consumed food normally equaled less than one pound.

Our heartfelt condolences to the poor women who restricted fat intake for seven years – they must have felt like crap. That's a great deal of sacrifice for one lousy pound and no health improvement.

You know what we call this? A waste of valuable time and energy.

Women are constantly told to reduce fat and slim down for another reason: breast cancer. But Harvard researcher Karin Michels found women who were overweight or obese at age eighteen had a 43 percent *less* chance of developing breast cancer than women in lower weight categories. Yes, those who weighed more were *less* susceptible to breast cancer. You don't hear your doctor pressuring you to gain weight early on so you don't get breast cancer, do you? The SBM is clear: "Eating fat and being fat is bad." Any research to the contrary goes right out the window.

If restricting fats doesn't help you lose weight, live longer, avoid cancer, or prevent heart attacks, why do we allow ourselves to be spoon-fed this garbage? To the health police and other skinny bitches near and far, we say, "Shut up about making us feel guilty every time we enjoy foods that are high in fat!" Promoting the myth that fat is bad is not intelligent. This is not a research finding, it's a cultural catastrophe. Gary Taubes wonderfully summed it up in his 2001 *Science* article: "Fifty years and hundreds of millions of dollars of research have failed to prove that low-fat diets will help you live longer."

CARB CENTRAL

If low-fat isn't the answer, then it has to be low-carb, right? But the Women's Health Initiative also studied the effects of a high-carbohydrate, low-fat eating pattern. The result? Eating high-carb didn't increase body weight, triglycerides, or other heart disease indicators, nor did it lead to increased risk of diabetes through blood glucose or insulin levels in women.

(Yes, we'll happily butter our bread, thank you.)

We know this may be counterintuitive to everything you were raised to believe in your home, at the doctor's office, or in health class. And some parents, teachers, and health-care providers may shoot back with, "Well, if the research has failed to prove in all these years that eating low-fat/low-carb is the best thing for you, then we just need to do more research so we can prove it."

Our society may be slow to catch up with the research, but you don't have to be. Take note of the sources listed in the back of this book and dive into your own research. Even if eating a low-fat, low-carb, and low-calorie diet *was* good for you, we found more proof that dieting is one of the biggest failures around.

Some of the most intriguing findings revolve around teens, such as the 2007 *Project EAT-II (Eat Among Teens)* study and a 2003 report in *Pediatrics*. These studies use a cool research method called a longitudinal design. This kind of research is long-term and follows people over time. When researchers study the same people over time, they discover the actual causes of behavior.

These studies researched thousands of dieting teens and preteens, and the discoveries were sobering. One group of children weighed themselves frequently, worried about their weight, and forced themselves to eat less. Across a five-year time span, this group of teens actually *gained* more weight than other teens. Yes, dieting actually *caused* weight gain. Poor kids. They were trying so hard to lose weight and be thin. We live in a world that promotes low-fat, low-calorie, and low-carb, remember? Dieting is encouraged. No one really thinks teens should diet. But they do think overweight teens should make "lifestyle changes" and "watch what they eat." You know, like going on a diet, but *never* getting off of it, which is exactly what these teens are trying to do. That's the clear message they receive. But are those kids actually enjoying their lives? Are they happy? No, the studies show they wasted their time dieting, because they thought they shouldn't eat "bad" foods. They were ashamed of their

---

[2] Most of the studies we cite in this book are longitudinal, because this type of research can actually prove causation. If you've taken a course in statistics, then you know correlation does not prove causation.

bodies, their eating, and themselves.

At the five-year follow up, the teens in this study gained fifteen more pounds than the non-dieters. Perhaps a well-meaning doctor or parent told them they were too fat; they needed to lose weight for their health. But that advice obviously did more harm than good, judging from the outcome. Everyone is on the bandwagon to "identify the overweight child." Why? So he or she can try to restrict his calories, fats, and carbohydrates? What will be the outcome? Restrictive and erratic eating CAUSES WEIGHT GAIN. It actually slows down body functions, including metabolism.

How could such well-intentioned plans go awry? Simple. Dieters become entirely too hungry to control their eating, and over time they travel into the land of binge-eating. Denying themselves pleasurable foods, even in moderation, seems to awaken an inner rebel. Dieters miss forbidden foods so much – perhaps foods their teachers, doctors, or parents told them they just shouldn't eat – that they eventually go overboard with those forbidden foods. And then SHAME arrives on the doorstep. "You shouldn't have eaten so much!" it scolds, or "What's wrong with you?" The dieter may even hear these statements from a friend or family member. Either way, they're left with an overwhelming feeling of humiliation and failure, locked in a world where they feel fat – and totally responsible for it. They just can't seem to get it right.

But don't you see? The dieter didn't fail. It's the entire dieting mentality (Okay, fine – lifestyle change mentality). Thinking you'll be thin by cutting back on calories, carbs, and fats is a set-up for failure.

Why do weight trackers gain the most weight? Maybe they are the ones who don't eat their breakfast. We know people who eat breakfast are more likely to control their weight than people who don't. But who's likely to skip breakfast? Dieters struggling to lose weight. Gee, we were all told if we eat less, it's better, right? Perhaps skipping breakfast makes dieters feel they're doing the proper thing for weight control. After all, they notice their stomachs become flatter and suddenly they feel more in control – thinner – as if they've earned a gold star on their diets. But still, those who skip breakfast wind up weighing more than those who chow down.

We say: Eat your breakfast! It's the best way to manage your weight, and besides that, breakfast provides the energy you need at the beginning of your day.

Here's another major reason dieting causes weight gain: no food = no energy.

Dieting teens in the *Project EAT-II* study had *decreased* physical activity by the time of the five-year follow up. The effect was even stronger for dieting boys, who typically require even more calories than girls do during adolescence.

Hello! Our bodies require food for energy, just as a car needs gas. Have you ever run out of gas? Your car just sits there. You can yell at it and get angry, but without gas it isn't going to budge. Food is fuel for the body. Shut up, and fuel yourself! The teens in the study were so hungry they didn't have enough energy to move around and exercise.

Pressure from society to cut back on food has created a troubling ripple effect. Millions of people, especially vulnerable children and teens still developing their physical bodies, *and* their identities, have been robbed of both nutrition and self-esteem.

Dieting is an epic FAIL.

FOOD FOR THOUGHT

Being too thin can be dangerous to your health. Everybody seems to agree that being overweight may be a major health risk, but several studies – including one published in 2006 in the *New England Journal of Medicine* – point out that being underweight can also shorten your life span. Somehow the part about underweight people being unhealthy never generated buzz.

The health police always want us to lose more weight. (More, more, more!) While many medical experts continue to cram the thinness ideal down our throats, some smart cookies, like the American Diabetes Association, actually pass along the truth – which shows an overweight person needs to lose only 5 to 10 percent of their total body weight to dramatically improve their health. Most people are told they can always improve their health by becoming as thin as they can – "you can never be too thin," right? – but this is unnecessary.

Seriously?

It's true.

In 1999, the *New England Journal of Medicine* suggested, "... for seriously overweight persons, the range of healthy weights is often practically unachievable. However, reductions of even 4 to 10 percent of weight can substantially improve blood pressure, serum lipid levels, and glucose tolerance and can reduce the incidence of diabetes and hypertension."

Don't you think it's time to stop setting your weight goals so high? (Make that low.) Unattainable goals set you up for failure. If health reasons are the real motivation behind your desire to hit that weight goal, then understand you don't need to reach the thinnest possible weight range to have terrific health benefits. So, chill out and change your lifestyle – just a bit – by *not* dieting. You'll then be able to stop binge-eating and gradually increase your activity levels. You'll naturally drop a few pounds *and* drop a huge load from your psyche. You'll stop hating yourself and not constantly feel like a failure. After you succeed with your new goals of eating well, not bingeing, and increasing your activity level, then when someone advises you to lose even more weight, feel free to tell them, "SHUT UP and BACK OFF."

A great deal of evidence indicates a sedentary lifestyle may be the *real* contributor to health statistics. Many researchers who conclude that excess weight leads to health issues haven't included fitness levels in their studies. However, several studies show exercise level is a strong, independent predictor of health indicators such as heart disease and cancer. Take the 1999 *Aerobic Center Longitudinal* study, which concluded, "Low fitness level was an independent predictor of mortality in overweight, obese, and normal weight men."

This is good news, because it reminds us we can do something *fun*; something we *can* control, to take care of our health.

THE POWER OF LOVE

Fat phobia reigns supreme. You can find evidence of this in almost any magazine or on most TV talk shows. Just look at the headlines that sport the same messages: "Watch what you eat!" "Cut back on carbs!" "Eat low-fat!" We are constantly inundated with the belief that we need to be thin to be healthy. It dominates our attention so much we've overlooked astounding research revealing the best ingredient for glowing health: Happiness.

But no one cares if you're happy, right? Just don't be fat.

In 2010, Columbia University Medical Center reported that people with *positive affect* – viewing the glass half full instead of half empty – had significantly less risk of heart disease across a ten-year longitudinal study. Joy, happiness, excitement, enthusiasm, and contentment have a protective effect on heart disease. This effect was so powerful that even when people went through a period of depression, it had no impact on their overall health. They still maintained an underlying positive attitude and benefited from its protection against heart disease. Simply put, happier people are healthier, and they live longer than others.

All of this made us think. Why do physicians insist on harping about our weight instead of encouraging us to be happy, or even improve our love lives?

Psychological factors greatly impact heart disease – those who will die from it versus those who recover. Depression, anxiety, hopelessness, hostility, and anger have all been linked to higher cardiac mortality rates, making death 1.5 to 2.5 times more likely for people with these specific emotional difficulties. If you're lonely, have significant family conflict, or don't get enough emotional support, this severely increases your risk of heart disease and stroke. But maybe it's just easier to restrict the fats you eat? Shut up about that. If you care about your health, you can't ignore the emotional areas in your life. Face it. You may have to do some emotional digging and uncover core issues that are holding you back and keeping you stuck.

Bottom line: we all need love, fulfillment, and happiness.

Are you bitter? Can't forgive? Holding a grudge? Let it go. Or is it just easier to cut back on carbs? Anger and hostility play a vital role in heart disease. We're told to "let go and forgive." True, it may not be easy at times, but when you take a hard look at any resentments you're holding on to, and then become open to working through and releasing them, you actually feed yourself a powerful nutrient.

There's more. We found two other factors linking emotions to heart disease. The first revolves around people who feel they have little or no control at work. These folks have a greater risk for heart disease and death. The second focuses on women who are caregivers – that is, women who care for their children twenty-one hours a week or more, or their grandchildren, or an ill spouse for nine hours a week or more. These women have double the risk for heart disease compared to women without caregiving responsibilities.

If you feel you have little control over your job, examine your situation and consider other options. And to all you caregiving women (and men) out there, let's get you some support. How about more help at home so you can get your workouts in? It's vital to create time each day to check in and take care of yourself. Your life may depend on it.

SHUT UP, AND MAKE LOVE

If you truly want to cut your chances of heart disease, you'll love the 2010 *American Journal of Cardiology* report about a sixteen-year study that discovered men (ages forty to seventy) who had sex twice a week or more reduced their risk of heart attack by 50 percent. The physical and emotional effects of sex protect our heart health. The analysis took into account other risk factors such as age, weight, blood pressure, and cholesterol levels. Nice. And making love has also been known to reduce prostate cancer, boost the immune system, and reduce the chances of catching colds and flu. Don't you love it?

HIDDEN MORSELS

We were worried that fat-phobic America wouldn't hear about the cool 2006 Swedish research concerning weight and heart disease, so we're serving it up here.

One study looked at twelve thousand people who suffered a heart attack. Those who lost weight afterward had a lower survival rate. And those who gained weight were, as one researcher noted, "none the worse for it, even if they were overweight from the start." Research director Ronnie Willenheimer reported, "European recommendations state that overweight patients after myocardial infarction (heart attack) should be recommended to lose weight. But the recommendations are not based on any studies, because our study is, in fact, the first in the field. And it unfortunately indicates that medical science may have shortened the lives of number of overweight patients with myocardial infarction by persuading them to diet."

He also states that weight loss after a heart attack "should not be viewed as a welcome joy. It may mean the patient is sicker than previously thought."

The second Swedish study looked at fifty thousand people in an attempt to see if obesity was a risk factor for heart disease. The research concluded that obesity, without other risk factors, didn't create a higher risk for a heart attack. Sixteen percent of obese people didn't smoke, have diabetes, high blood pressure, or high blood lipids. Obesity by itself, without these other risk factors, didn't increase the risk for heart attack. The study found obesity increased the risk of heart attack only for single men who lived alone and were self-employed or working class.

Does your heart doctor tell you to lose weight? According to this study, your physician should be advising you to find a roommate and get a new job. Our recommendations: rather than trying to starve yourself healthy, try dating, or set up a cool job interview. Shut up, and live a little!

Yes, the best alternative to dieting is happiness. The best thing you can do is get happy. Now is good. You can start by not bitching. Think about it; how much progress can you make in moving any part of your life forward when you're constantly harping on yourself and others?

PUTTING IT ALL TOGETHER

Since super low-fat/low-calorie/low-carb isn't the way to go, what is the recipe for success?

First, let's try increasing our intake of fresh fruits and vegetables. That always works. This is healthy, easy, and worth your investment. Receiving a good balance of all food groups is vital for overall health. [See Chapter Three.] A great deal of evidence demonstrates getting enough sleep is strongly related to your good health, and also ties into weight maintenance. If we can lose weight in our sleep, we're all for it. Finally, physical exercise is the undisputed king of good health (as long as you take care of your body with enough food from all of the food groups).

Think of it as a recipe. Take eating from all food groups, especially the neglected fruits and veggies, mix that with getting enough sleep and a reasonable amount of vigorous, enjoyable exercise, and you'll be sure to experience great success. All of this works together without diminishing your self-esteem or making you feel like a failure.

Embrace this: *You* are responsible for the events and conditions you bring into your life. It's that simple. You can either force-feed the SBM – a mindset that only lets you feel good about yourself when you starve and are skinny – or you can open the refrigerator door of life and enjoy the smorgasbord. Do the latter more often and, surprise!

You won't be a bitch.

Whenever we're caught up with dieting, equating being skinny with success, and watching what we eat for fear we'll be fat and unhealthy, we overlook something obvious when it comes to the most vital muscle we have to nourish: our hearts.

The lesson? Make progress toward creating that *positive affect*. And don't diet! Look at it this way: remember all the energy it took to actually go on a diet and stay on a diet? Marvel at yourself for a moment. If you actually had enough energy to do *that*, all for the sake of good health, then certainly you have the energy to direct your attention to something more substantial. Take all the life force you used to avoid eating everything from an extra Saltine to a teaspoon of salad dressing, and channel that energy into enjoying and appreciating all the good things in your life. Let the skinny bitches enjoy their non-fat tofu chai lattes. Instead, go ahead, dip your hand into the cookie jar of life – and love yourself for doing so.

Shut Up, And Don't Even Touch Our Chocolate!

A 2010 study of 19,000 people in Germany
found that people who ate the highest amounts
of chocolate had lower blood pressure and a
39 percent lower risk of having a heart attack
or stroke. The group most protected by
eating chocolate ate about a bar a week — or
one-sixth of a bar per day. And, no, health freaks,
it wasn't just dark chocolate. It worked for
all types of chocolate. The cocoa has flavonoids
that are heart-healthy. So go ahead, make your day
and consume that yummy chocolate.

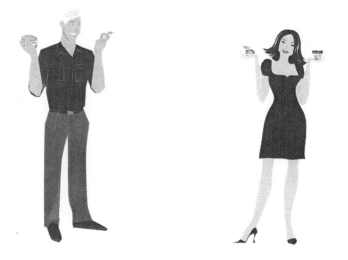

*"Life's a banquet and most poor suckers
are starving to death."*

—Auntie Mame

Chapter Three
Follow Your Hunger

THE LEGENDARY CHARACTER AUNTIE MAME had it right: There's
no time like right now. So, take a big bite out of life – all parts of
life, including eating. Yes, you can avoid the chronic dieting cycle by
simply following your hunger. Note these guidelines and allow the
transformation to happen.

1. Embrace the revamped Food Pyramid.
2. Get back in touch with your body's natural hunger and fullness
   cues.
3. Chuck your list of good and bad foods.
4. Avoid making food choices out of fear. When you eat
   everything in moderation, food has no power over you.

FOOD PYRAMID REDUX

This isn't a headscratcher. There's a good reason the American
Dietetic Association suggests following the revamped 1992 Food
Pyramid, now dubbed MyPyramid. It works, because this is the most

effective way to manage optimal health. All foods can be included in MyPyramid, so you have no foods to fear or avoid. (We know, we're so programmed to fear some foods, this seems too good to be true.)

MyPyramid, which was set into place in 2005, is similar to the old Food Pyramid but it is tossed on its side. The new model suggests that for optimal health we need to incorporate healthy portions of *all* food groups in our everyday food plan – fruits, vegetables, dairy, protein, fat, and carbohydrates. Yes, they include fats. Yes, they list carbs. What's the problem? Why are fats and carbs despised by so many? We're brainwashed into thinking they're evil, creating tremendous pressure to avoid these two essential food groups.

Here's a *quick* glance at each food group and its importance.

Carbohydrates. They're your friend, so shut up and eat some. Say hello to whole grains, bread, cereal, fruits, veggies, and pasta. Carbs are simply energy/fuel your body needs for physical activity. Carbs are also vital in helping your organs function properly. Organs – you know, your heart, your brain? As we all know by now, grains high in fiber and low in sugar are healthier. They assist with weight maintenance and regulate healthy blood sugar levels. Consume them. But don't berate yourself when you eat non-whole-wheat carbs. Remember: when you fear certain foods and try to avoid them, suppressed cravings for those foods will eventually stalk you like a modern-day blood sucker from *True Blood*. Before you know it, you could find yourself hiding in the basement secretly munching on those damn Cocoa Puffs you've been avoiding all week. Being at war with your hunger isn't necessary. Remember, everything in moderation. That's the key to overcoming eating disorders and breaking free from a world of food phobias. So, tell the Carb Nazis to step aside while you enjoy a nice plate of pasta.

Still cranky about carbs? Did you know carbs play a role in depression? Many mood swingers deprive themselves of carbs, then later binge on them, not realizing carb cravings have a great deal to do with the body's natural chemistry. Your body breaks down carbs into serotonin, a form of anti-depressant. Yeah, so maybe the reason you got so depressed in the first place had something to do with not consuming enough simple and complex carbs.

According to the Harvard School of Public Health, "No one knows the long-term effects of eating little or no carbohydrates." And really – why should you be the guinea pig?

Still hate carbs? Get over it.

Fruits and vegetables. Obviously fruits and veggies contain multiple vitamins and minerals and come in a variety of colors, each offering different antioxidants used by the body. Choose from the rainbow spectrum of fruits and veggies. No one can dispute the extraordinary impact of these food groups on your health, so enjoy. Even dried fruit is a plus.

Dairy. Milk and other calcium-rich foods are essential for optimal health. In fact, dairy products contain valuable nutrients, including protein, potassium, phosphorus, and vitamins A and D. Dairy products are calcium-rich and an excellent way to give your body the required calcium it needs to build, and maintain, healthy bones. According to the International Osteoporosis Foundation, other calcium-rich foods include eggs, broccoli, apricots, tofu, red kidney beans, pasta, salmon, white rice, macaroni and cheese, and pizza. What are the chances of white rice and mac 'n' cheese sitting near each other on a list of healthy foods?

You probably won't feel motivated to embrace calcium if we tell you eighty-year-olds can get osteoporosis. But take note. Around the age of thirty, women become unable to store large amounts of calcium and need to rely on what they've already stored in their bodies. So, shake yourself out of that Skinny Bitches Mindset, because you don't have your entire life to store calcium. Your risk for stress fractures, and even broken hips, rises with severe calcium deficits. Dieting and other eating problems can cause extreme problems in the bones of young people. Actually, according to a 2005 report in the *International Journal of Epidemiology*, consuming dairy products helps decrease the incidence of stroke, heart disease, colon cancer, breast cancer, type 2 diabetes, hypertension, and insulin resistance.

Yes, contrary to some beliefs, dairy is actually cool. (Excuse us while we wipe off our milk mustaches.)

Protein. In the 1980s, avoiding protein was a diet fad, but you can't even build lean muscle without this nutrient. Your body uses protein for your skin, hair, nails, tendons, and cartilage and it aids circulation, tissue repair, and healing from injury. Proteins are found in many sources, including tofu, beans, peas, nuts, dairy, eggs, fish, and meat. There are twenty-two different amino acids, which are the building blocks for protein. A *complete protein* contains all the amino acids needed by the body. Eating a variety of protein sources increases your likelihood of receiving and benefitting from all twenty-two amino acids. People who completely avoid eggs, meat, and/or dairy have a difficult time consuming all the amino acids the body requires. Since our bodies can't store protein, we need to put it into our diets throughout the day.

Don't let anyone fool you. Getting enough protein and calcium in your diet while abstaining from eating meat, fish, eggs, or dairy products is extremely difficult. Vegetarians and vegans need to take extra care and watch for nutritional deficits. Veganism and vegetarianism aren't the only healthy lifestyles, and if you aren't informed about how to obtain enough protein, calcium, and iron, these eating regimens aren't healthy. And hey – vegans and veggies. We dig you, so we're not in the mood to meet you in a back alley for a fencing match with carrot sticks. We just want to make sure everyone receives everything they need from their diets. And yeah – we're talking to you, too, meat-phobics. You have the same needs as the rest of us. But you may be in denial. Perhaps some skinny bitches failed to explain about the twenty-two amino acids and the difference between complete and incomplete proteins. Bottom line: stop shorting yourself on a variety of high quality proteins, including meat, carb, dairy, and vegetable sources.[3]

---

[3] We're jazzed by Michael Murray's *Healing Foods*/2005, which offered an in-depth look at each amino acid and where it's found.

While many people become vegans or vegetarians because they're animal lovers or believe we shouldn't consume animals, some veggies use this as a way to cut out more *bad* groups of food, mostly to feed an eating disorder. Be honest about your motivation.

Fat. And finally, a few words about our little friend fat. Think of it as the satiety nutrient, because fat causes us to feel more satisfied from meal to meal so we don't binge. Ironic, isn't it? The two most feared and avoided food groups – fat and carbs – are the two that help protect us from bingeing.

Many people are caught up in a cycle of avoiding carbs and fats as part of a restrictive food plan, then binge on them later. In fact, avoiding those food groups *causes* bingeing. And what's life without Cheetos and Oreos (in moderation of course)? Our friend fat also promotes beautiful skin, hair, and nails. Even more importantly, fat surrounds and protects our organs, including the brain and heart.

YOUR HUNGER CUES

Out: dieting.

In: eating.

During your dieting journey, perhaps you've lost the ability to know when you're hungry and when you're full. You may even experience guilt when you're hungry and second-guess yourself about when you should eat. Worse, you may beat yourself up when you're full.

The good news? You can relearn how to be in touch with your body. You can listen to your internal hunger and fullness cues.

The first thing to do is eat, as in three meals a day and two to three snacks a day. Take that action and you'll recreate a habit of eating regularly. Now, don't have a fit. We know you're not accustomed to someone telling you to eat, but we suggest that whenever you eat, rate your hunger from zero to ten. You should eat when you reach a six or seven (out of ten) on your perceived hunger scale. No, not a nine or ten. You shouldn't wait until you're famished. Eating too late sets you up to overeat and feeds into the cycle you're trying to break.

When you eat, keep track of how full you become. Try to stop at about six, or seven (out of ten). With this new plan of eating before you're famished, you'll begin to eat less hurriedly so you actually taste your food again. This will help you enjoy food and break out of destructive eating cycles.

Watch for two psychological issues that often come up with the "eat when you're hungry/stop when you're full" plan: fear and fullness.

If you have a great deal of fear about eating, these feelings may throw off the accuracy of rating your hunger and fullness. You might get full quickly because you're worried about what you're eating. Or you may not have any idea how to tell when you're hungry. Your body may have temporarily stopped giving you a hunger signal, because you rarely listen to it. If hunger and fullness are too confusing for you right now, then use more mechanical eating methods until your body's natural hunger and fullness signals are working again. This means eating three healthy meals a day, plus good snacks. Smaller amounts of any foods you like are fine snacks. Snacks help keep your blood sugar and energy level more even throughout the day, and they can stop your hunger from reaching out of control levels by the time you have a meal.

Constipation also interferes with hunger and fullness cues. Many chronic dieters have temporarily slowed their bodies' ability to process food. When they do eat, these folks frequently find themselves bloated and constipated, which makes them feel even fatter. This certainly influences how they perceive hunger and fullness. Constipation makes you feel less hungry and more full. Challenging, yes, because when you begin eating again, you may feel a little worse before you feel better. If you become constipated while you move away from restricting your food to consuming food on regular basis, take note:

— Do Not Use Laxatives Under Any Circumstances —

Laxatives work by stripping the lower colon of waste that was going to be eliminated anyway. The colons of some chronic dieters are so stripped from using and abusing laxatives they no longer function properly. So, since adult diapers aren't in style this season, you need to realize erratic and restrictive eating is the core problem and that eating regularly again, over time, will allow you to have regular bowel movements.

You'll feel better once your body is processing food again. Receiving enough fiber in your diet always helps, especially from nutrient-rich fruits and veggies. Consume these regularly. Don't forget that exercise will help restore your body's natural rhythm of regular movement – even just going for a walk. Some people do require medical intervention for chronic constipation. If this problem develops, you will want to work with a physician who has knowledge of eating disorders.

THE GOOD FOODS/BAD FOODS MYTH

In the quest to have a healthy relationship with your body and food, consider giving up your rigid list of good foods and bad foods. Good foods are things you consider healthy to eat and you don't feel guilty about consuming. You know what we mean – lettuce, carrots, tomatoes, tofu. When you stick to these so-called safe food choices, at the end of the day, you say to yourself, "I did well today."

Bad foods, like cake, cookies, pasta, ice cream, and French fries tend to actually taste good. These are the foods you think you shouldn't eat – they contain too many calories, too many carbs, too much sugar, and so on.

For "successful" dieters, the Good Food lists becomes shorter and shorter over time, and the Bad Food list grows. The problem is, this restriction reduces your quality of life, because food choices become too rigid and narrow. You can't appreciate life the way you naturally would; you either avoid foods on the list, or lose control and binge on them. "If I'm going to indulge in one of the foods from the dark side," you reason, "I should totally give in and eat a massive quantity, since I won't be seeing it again anytime soon."

Unfortunately, when you binge, you eat so fast you can't savor or enjoy the taste of the food anyway.

Write down your list of Good Foods and Bad Foods. (Do it right now. We'll wait...)

Now, rewrite your lists of how feared the food is. Rate your Bad Foods from zero (No Fear) to one hundred (Freaking Out of Your Skin/Would Never Eat It!). Start reincorporating these feared foods back into your diet. Begin with lower-ranked Freak-Out foods first, then move up the ranks on the Freak Out Meter over time. Put the tasty foods you love back into your diet and guess what? There's nothing to bitch about.

Twenty-one-year-old Tifani, who recovered from an eating disorder and years of brainwashing herself to an "eat right" life, tells us...

> 66 Any time I tried to eat low-fat, low-carb, or any other type of diet that caused me to restrict or remove a specific food group, I found myself wanting that food group more. It became obsessive thinking for me. I would say, "Oh, I'm going to cut this out because it's bad for me" and then all I wanted to eat was that food, which would end with me bingeing on it. THERE IS NO SUCH THING AS GOOD AND BAD FOOD! All food is good in moderation. It was hard for me to learn this because I grew up with a mom who had rigid ideas of good and bad foods. As I experimented with eating all sorts of food and seeing what my body did with them, I truly learned that my body – and everyone's bodies – process a piece of cake and a piece of buttered toast the same way – as the food pyramid exchanges of a grain and a fat. If I only eat cake for breakfast, lunch, and dinner, it's bad for me. However, if I eat only eat toast it's bad for me as well. It's all about balance. 99

NOTHING TO FEAR

Think about this: when your food is broken into categories of good and bad, it has too much power over you. Instead of following your hunger and embracing what tastes good, you're fearful and riddled with shame about the very thing your body needs to survive: FOOD! When you conquer your Bad Food list and move them into a Safe Zone, you'll notice food no longer has a stranglehold on you. You'll be free to follow your hunger, eat food you love, and never have to binge, because you'll always have enough of all the foods you want.

Learning to estimate healthy portion sizes is the next skill you need to learn to maintain a healthy weight without trying so hard. The Food Pyramid will guide you on correct portions while you're a rookie. But when you get your hunger and fullness cues back, you won't need to worry about portion sizes, because you'll always know how to stop eating when you're full.

When in doubt, keep this in mind. When it comes to eating, never, ever let fear be your guide. Remember, everything in moderation.

Shut Up, And Stop Perpetuating Skinny Myths

Myth: When you're dead, all you want people to say is, "Boy, was she skinny!" or "Damn, did he have a hot body!"

Fact: *Deep down, you want to live your life fully and leave behind a legacy.* If you waste all of your energy trying to be skinny, you'll miss the true meaning of life and understanding your true purpose.

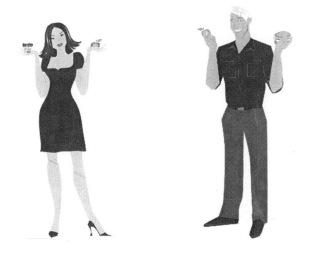

"There is no giant step or magic pill that does it.
It's all about taking small steps."

—Gilad

Chapter Four
The Thing About Exercise

HERE'S THE THING ABOUT EXERCISE: Do some.

True, exercising may seem like a simple task, but who hasn't stumbled on that path? Life, circumstances, and things in general always get in the way. So does the media. After all, the media loves flooding us with images of perfection. Like we need to look and act a certain way if we want to fit in. Yeah, we understand being liked is a common desire, but none of us can advance our health objectives if we're always striving to morph into unrealistic images of skinny bitches – most of whom have been photoshopped. (Ahem ... thanks, Ralph Lauren.) Inevitably, we end up beating ourselves up because our body image and weight goals are unrealistic. Unless you really want to be forever hungry and neurotic, stop striving to look perfect by indulging in a restrictive, snarky Skinny Bitches Mindset (SBM). We suspect the SBM lifestyle isn't your choice. Snarky doesn't feed the soul.

So, when it comes to exercise, shut up about restricting your eating. Besides, if you choose starvation and/or severe food restriction, you won't have the energy to exercise anyway.

Do you folks remember that bestseller *Do What You Love, The Money Will Follow* by Marsha Sinetar? In a nutshell Marsha tells us the people who follow their hearts and perform work they love will be blessed with a sweet financial flow. This is basic physics, baby. Align your thoughts in a positive direction and you'll experience positive things in life, right? As within, so without.

So, when it comes to exercise, we're here to tell you: Do what you love and the body will follow.

Translation: Don't over think exercise. Just have fun doing it.

In addition to being a professional writer, Greg has moonlighted as a certified fitness instructor for more than fifteen years. He's taught a wide variety of classes, from aerobics and body sculpting to weight training and cycle spin classes. Greg meets happy people in those fitness rooms, because most are doing activities they love, which makes their fitness regime fun. And isn't fun what exercise is supposed to be about?

Think back to when you were a kid. You played outside with your friends, ran around the backyard, rode a bike, ran around in the park, swam, and enjoyed games like tag and jump rope. We propose you already know what kind of exercise you love to do, or would like to do. And good Lord, there's such variety – dance (we dig Zumba), weight training, cycling, aerobics, kick-boxing, hiking, jogging, mountain climbing, swimming. What works for you? Which one works for your body? Experiment. Pick something and try it.

But take note: cross training is your friend.

So far in this book, we've promoted eating and eating well versus restricting food intake. The same advice applies to exercise. Common sense tells you to feed your body *activity*, and the more variety, the better. That's cross training.

Many athletes cross train with different types of activity and exercise during a set time period, rather than repeating the same activities. Why does this work? For starters, it keeps your body – your muscles – guessing, meaning, they're working and adapting more frequently to the kind of workout you're doing. When you stick with only one kind of exercise regime, your body lands on a plateau where it becomes accustomed to what you're doing and stalls. Your muscles are looking for new challenges. The plateau effect can happen as early as six weeks, or after several months of consistent exercise. That's when your body is asking you to work something new into your workout regime.

If your workout is mostly cardio, then consider adding body sculpting with weights – even light weights – to the mix. If you're doing body sculpting or weight training, then add cardio. You get the picture. The idea is to move around and have fun. The more you can tap into you're playful side, the better off you'll be. You're moving around because, well, it's natural. Don't turn it into a major task you'll bitch about later. Your attitude matters, so try exercising with a positive mindset. Afterward, pause to gauge how you feel. Does it stimulate you? If you're sore or injured, turn things down a notch.

Are you hitting roadblocks to success in this area? Plateaus are common, and even expected. We'd never propose you "get off your fat ass and make it happen" like some other diet manifestos do. That's because this isn't a diet manifesto. But if you're stuck, you're stuck. Let's look at that. Here's a list of excuses we hear from people who tell themselves they can't exercise.

The Excuse: "I'm too busy!"
What We Say: *Welcome to time management and prioritizing.*
Action: Shut up and have fun. Open your monthly calendar and schedule exercise time. If you can book a meeting with a skinny little bitch client, you can book a meeting with yourself.

The Excuse: "I'm tired!"

What We Say:	*Shut up and wake up.* Exercising increases your energy, period. And guess what? You'll be less tired over time.
Action:	Look at your sleep habits. Are you getting enough rest each night to sustain healthy physical activity? Now, notice your eating plan. Are you eating enough fats, carbs, and proteins to sustain your energy, or is restricting food draining your life force?
The Excuse:	"I'm bored with my workout!"
What We Say:	*Shut up and change it!*
Action:	You wouldn't read the same book over and over, would you? Consider new forms of exercise you can add to your core routine. Think of it as sprinkling hot red peppers onto your pasta instead of Parmesan flakes.
The Excuse:	"This doesn't burn enough calories."
What We Say:	*Talking burns calories, but in this case, Shut up.*
Action:	Don't freak out over calorie-burning. You don't need to nickel and dime everything. Just have fun exercising. Trust us. Having fun is good for you.
The Excuse:	"I have nothing to wear."
What We Say:	*Shut up and put on your workout clothes.*
Action:	If you truly don't have anything to wear, here's a wild idea – go shopping and buy workout clothes. Just wear something comfortable. And if your gym feels like a Barbie and Ken fashion show, then go somewhere else.
The Excuse:	"Gym memberships are too pricey."
What We Say:	*Shut up and open your wallet.* Not *all* gym memberships are expensive, and you don't have to join a gym to be active.

Action:	Review possible outlets for activity and make good decisions based on your budget. And consider other outlets. There's yoga (from Bikram to Vinyasna), swimming, dance classes, cycling, and more. If finances are a concern, check out your local community colleges. Most have fitness classes and workout rooms at affordable rates for a semester or quarter. And don't forget to honestly check in with yourself. What are your priorities? Add up how much you spend at Starbucks, or its equivalent, each month. Then honestly ask yourself whether you still think you can't afford a gym or class membership, if that's something you truly want.
The Excuse:	"I don't like the way I look, and I feel ashamed when people see me work out."
What We Say:	*We understand.* So listen to us, sweetheart. You're beautiful and you look fine. Let's put it this way. Shame is not a natural feeling. It's learned. Underneath the shame is *you* – all you in all your splendor. There is nothing wrong with you. Let's say it again. *There is nothing wrong with you.* At times, you may feel the opposite is true, but the opposite can never really be true. *There is nothing wrong with you.* Shame is learned. And it can be unlearned.
Action:	Think of ways to find increased emotional support for your workouts, such as a workout buddy, someone to check in with. Plan ahead to reward yourself for meeting your goals. After one workout, treat yourself to something you love, such as a movie or a massage. Don't make food the reward.

STILL TRAPPED?

But what if you, like many people, feel trapped in your body – as if it's a prison? You feel alienated from your own body. Perhaps you cancel plans because, on a particular day, you don't feel your body is up to par and you don't want to be seen in public. Sometimes you dig a big old hole for yourself, so huge you can't even exercise at all. You feel too vulnerable and can't connect to your body through exercise. Know this: physical exercise is part of a healing journey, offering you a chance to reconnect with your body and establish a relationship that's compassionate, caring, and respectful. If your shame issues get in the way of living a full, productive life, take steps to transform that mindset – by exercising.

Depending upon the extent of your shame, consider joining a support group or seeing a counselor. Or perhaps you can have open, meaningful conversations with real friends who are committed to your well-being. Creating a network of support is always a good move. Here's the thing: unless you're an infant, no one is going to take care of you. We can cry about it, but at the end of the day, it's up to each of us to take care of ourselves, inside and out. If fiery internal dialogues stall your fitness endeavors, there's a way to move through that. You're not alone and *Nothing Is Wrong With You*. You can work it out.

What really works when it comes to exercise?

We suggest a good dose of cardio, mixed with body sculpting, during the course of each week. Here's why. We like to see you sweat – literally. And honestly, don't you feel better when you do? Don't you feel as if you're working your body hard and getting somewhere? You know why? Because you are. Perspiration is where it's at. Sweat. Don't just lift a few weights and call it a day. Push yourself a little. Don't be afraid to perspire.

Perspiration indicates you're working your heart, the most vital muscle in your body. When exercising, it's safest to start slow and increase the intensity over time. An out-of-shape person going out to shovel heavy snow in the driveway is *not* a good idea. Begin slowly and be satisfied with gradual progress. If you've been sedentary for awhile, make sure your doctor is comfortable with your exercise plan.

The best news of all? Regular physical activity can reduce your risk for cancer, heart disease, diabetes, and other chronic conditions. Significant studies on cardiovascular health show physical exercise is a strong predictor of heart fitness.

If you aren't doing so already, consider working out three to five times a week. You don't need to be sophisticated to find out how intense your workout should be. According to the Centers for Disease Control, the Borg's Rating of Perceived Exertion scale[4] is one way to measure the intensity level of your physical activity and estimate how hard your body is working. The Borg scale is correlated with your actual heart rate, so you can follow your body and adjust accordingly.

You don't need fancy equipment for a proper workout. You can rank your own exertion level and accurately know if your workout is too hard, too wimpy, or just right. Rate your level of exertion between 0 and 20 as you go through a workout. Nine is like a slow, comfortable walk, while 17 is challenging and you feel fatigue over time. Moderate intensity is a good goal to shoot for, with a perceived exertion rating of 12 to 13. For example, if you want to walk at a moderate level and rate your exertion at 19, that's your clue to back off to a slower, easier pace until you get back into the range you set for yourself. A length of 30 to 60 minutes per workout is recommended, several times per week. Over time, increasing your level of fitness will improve your body image. Doing something pro-active brings a great feeling of accomplishment.

Remember: skinny isn't the cure. You're not doing this to be skinny. You're exercising because it's good for you.

---

[4] View the Borg Rating on the U.S. government's web site: www.cdc.gov/physicalactivity/everyone/.../index.html

Consider mixing your workouts. At least every six weeks or so, add something new and ease off on other things. If you're a devotee of the treadmill, try the elliptical machine for twenty-five minutes, and then consider doing something like, say, walking up and down stairs for twelve to fifteen minutes. Or do some lunges. Most gyms have trainers to assist you, but make sure your trainer doesn't have the SBM and insists you must eat low-fat and low-carb to see results. Feel free to say, "Shut up!" if this happens.

For those of us who aren't active or haven't been active in a while, we're here to tell you what Greg often tells his spin classes: "Don't freak out!" Chances are you have exercised at one point or another in your life. If you found something you truly loved doing, gravitate in that direction. If all else fails, chuck frustration aside and start walking.

Yeah. It's true. Walking is one of the best forms of exercise, and the most natural. Consider going for long walks, as in more than a mile round trip. Build on that after two weeks, making it two miles, maybe three. If exercising truly rattles your nerves, it's okay – you can always walk. When all else fails, walk. The *Nurse's Health Study* (Willett, 1999) found that women who walked at a brisk pace for three or more hours per week were 30 to 40 percent less likely to have a heart attack compared to sedentary women. The effects equaled the results for more vigorous forms of physical activity. And it's never too late. Sedentary women who became active in middle age lowered their risk compared to those who remained sedentary.

Here's the thing – and you know this, we're just posting a reminder so you don't tumble down the cliff with society's other SBMers – exercise makes you naturally feel good. Your heart is pumping, your blood circulates. Basically darling, it's natural and good for you. We aren't meant to sit around and contemplate our navels all day long. Our bodies are designed to move. *Hello!* Why do you think we have them?

And don't forget to eat. (What a concept!) Your body requires nutrition before and after workouts. Check in for hunger and thirst cues. Create a habit of eating food and drinking plenty of water to re-hydrate yourself throughout the day. But keep in mind that after you exercise, your body will be looking to refuel and the best time frame to do this is before your body starts feeding itself off your muscle – within two hours after exercising.

We'll leave you with this. If you had a donkey pulling your cart, how would you treat it? Would you shout at the poor beast or use a whip to make it go? Would you starve it? Why do we think we need to treat our bodies like a poor ass? You should treat a living creature with nurturing and respect, especially when you want it to work for you. Do the same for yourself.

In the meantime, let's bust a few more myths.

MYTH BUSTING

Myth: "Nickel and Dime" thinking: "Well, if I ate French fries, that means I have to workout for 20 extra minutes!" Wrong!

Myth Buster: *"My goal is to workout three to five times a week* for at least forty-five to sixty minutes. Other than that, I just eat normally." Always try to get your workouts in, and always take care of your body with fluids and food. Burning the calories you eat through exercise is a tedious waste of time – and it's unnecessary.

Myth: "If I stay tied to the treadmill for an hour, I'm sure to lose weight."

Myth Buster: *Shut up and do activity that's vigorous,* fun, and makes you happy.

Myth: "I'll never get my workout done unless I kick my own ass."

Myth Buster: *You don't have to be mean to get yourself moving.*

Having a negative, punitive mindset about exercise will backfire and lead to a reduction in working out. When you feel like a failure, you give up. A little sugar will get you further than vinegar.

Myth: "I don't know how to exercise."

Myth Buster: *Don't underestimate yourself, honey.* If you can open your mouth to speak, you know how to exercise. Use your intuition. You *do* know how to exercise. You do it already without even knowing it. Learn to love your body again as you're being active. Choose internally driven activities. Don't be a rigid SBMer. Three words of wisdom to guide you: flexibility, moderation, and intuition.

Myth: "The more I exercise, the better shape I'll be in."

Myth Buster: *Not always the case.* Here's why: stress fractures and other injuries are common for people who over-exercise. In fact, too much exercise can wreak havoc on your body, your mind, and even your soul.

Jenni, a married thirty-four-year-old knitting aficionado tells us this chilling story.

> 66 When I was in the thick of things with my eating disorder, I showed up at the gym by 5 o'clock on most mornings. One day I looked across the gym and saw a woman who obviously had an eating disorder – she appeared thin, but not overly thin – whatever that means. But, it wasn't her size that caught my attention. It was her eyes. She had that crazed look of "I have to be here even though I hate it" while at the same time her expression seemed

dead. We stared at each other – not moving. After a few moments I realized I was staring into a huge mirror from across the room. Talk about a wake-up call. I was so disconnected from my own body that I didn't even recognize myself in a mirror! 99

Twenty-two-year old Erin shares how exercise can became a way to mask depression and other emotional problems.

66My roommate and I were already known as The Workout Roomies on campus, because we rose every morning at 5:45, before class, when the only other people in the gym were senior citizens. All the other students were still in bed. My roommate was able to keep this passion in check, but my exercise habits quickly spiraled out of control. I found myself adding runs around campus, second and third gym sessions each day, and crunches in my room during any free time I could find. Honestly, I had no social life because I was so busy trying to push away my depression through exercise. 99

In other words lovely people, sweat. But don't sweat it – please.

Soul Food

Do what you love, and the body will follow.

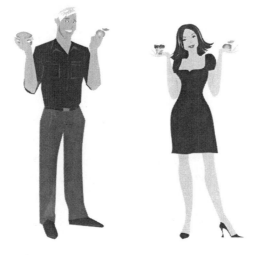

*"I finally realized that being grateful to my body
was key to giving more love to myself."*

—Oprah Winfrey, *O Magazine*

Chapter Five
Shut Up, About Hating Your Body

MIRROR, MIRROR ON THE WALL... Do you love what you see staring back at you in the mirror? Chances are you don't. According to the National Eating Disorders Association (NEDA), approximately 88 percent of females and 43 percent of males are dissatisfied with their bodies. Are we all that hideous? What's with all this hating?

The statistics are surprising. A landmark *Psychology Today* study in 1997 discovered people are so dissatisfied with their bodies that 24 percent of women and 17 percent of men would be willing to trade three years of their lives to accomplish their weight goals. Fifteen percent of women and 11 percent of men would trade five years of their lives to achieve their weight goals. Is the desire to be thin more precious than life itself?

Even our children aren't spared from self-hatred caused by the Skinny Bitches Mindset (SBM). A 2000 study found that 21 percent of five-year-olds were concerned about their weight and dissatisfied with their bodies. And in 2006, the *California Journal of Health*

Promotion revealed that by third, fourth, and fifth grades, 50 percent of children, both boys and girls, were dissatisfied with their size and shape. These are little kids! They should be enjoying themselves, not stressing about their size.

Wait – there's more. Even though dieting is an "epic fail," the habit persists: 25 percent of men, 45 percent of women, and 30 percent of middle-school girls are dieting on any given day. Thirty-five percent of dieters progress to pathological dieting (severely distressed, dieting chronically) and 25 percent of dieters will develop full-blown eating disorders. These statistics clearly indicate many people are locked into a lifetime of self-blame, low self-worth, and frustration. And since 85 to 95 percent of all dieters regain their weight within one to five years, each of these hard workers is set up to experience strong feelings of failure and shame.

Inga is a thirty-four-year-old photographer from Germany. For years, she's struggled with accepting herself and her body. She tells us...

66Not feeling at home in my body was my main problem. It's so easy nowadays to not like your body, especially if you're transforming into a teenager. All around you the media projects perfect faces and bodies. The most perfect bodies have the best lives and are the happiest people on the planet; only THEY are successful. That's the message you get if you follow today's advertisements or commercials. I remember feeling different about a lot of issues than girls my age. When we started to look at boys, I never understood it was always about body images, rather than characteristics or other features. I didn't like my body at all, mostly because I didn't feel I could fit into that mindset. I didn't want to be judged by just my body. But no one seemed interested in that idea. 99

It's time to stop hating our bodies.

The good news is, negative body image is something we all learned – and that means this mindset can be *unlearned*. That's right. Have you ever watched a baby or toddler examine his or her hands or feet with wonder, or sport a beautiful smile when grabbing fat on their body? We're all born with an innate affection for ourselves and our bodies. As we're taught that only thinness is beautiful, our eyes learn to hate what they see. The more unrealistic the images become, the more we believe we don't measure up. We can, to some degree, thank the advertising industry for this. The industry usually selects models from the thinnest 2 percent of the population. Their already-thin images are further elongated and shaved through Photoshop. No wonder many of us can't sleep at night – we can't stop thinking we're fat and unacceptable.

SEVEN WAYS TO STOP HATING YOUR BODY

1. Reframe Your Thinking

"If only I weighed X all my dreams would come true?" Does that sound familiar? What do you think would happen if you lost those inches or pounds and met your weight goals?

"I'll finally meet the right person," you say, or, "I'll finally have a great sex life!" or "Only then will people really be attracted to me!" People believe weight loss will magically spawn the right job, the right friends, popularity, financial success, good relationships—and more. Let's be real. How can losing weight automatically cure loneliness, boredom, poverty and self-esteem issues? Of course it doesn't. We absorb these fantasies from television shows, movies, and magazines. The irony is, most of us have actually achieved our goal weight at one time or another, and even though we had evidence our hopes and dreams didn't magically come true because we lost weight, we keep repeating the cycle.

Stop trying to solve all your problems through weight loss. Do you truly want people to love you because of your size? Ultimately, we all want to be loved and accepted for who we are.

So, ditch the "If only I weighed X" fantasy. Instead, make this your new mantra: "I choose to love and accept myself and all my dreams will be manifested, under grace." Now we're talking. Instead of trying to change and punish yourself, redirect that energy and feed your inner world something substantial. Make the choice. Refuse to hate yourself for any reason. And remember, stop thinking or believing every good thing in your life will happen if and when you become thinner.

2. Eradicate Body Perfectionism

Do you pick yourself apart in the mirror every day? Do you weigh yourself to see if you're good enough? Body perfectionists don't give themselves credit for positive things about their bodies. They may be able to jog long distances, they may have strong arms, lovely hair, or gorgeous eyes, but those things don't matter. The body perfectionist only sees negatives – and then it's search and destroy. Can you relate to any of this? If so, make a list of good things about your body, and feel free to enlist the help of friends and trusted family members if you get stuck on this one.

Next, set realistic goals. Begin by turning your perfectionist thinking upside down, because you'll never be satisfied with the goals that mindset creates. You may accomplish a great deal, but never meet your target of perfection. You'll always feel like a failure, no matter how much you do. So give yourself more credit. Set goals you can actually attain. Realistic goal setting will help you overcome perfectionism, improve your self-esteem, and accomplish even more. Remember: the decision to love and accept yourself and your body is all yours. Choose wisely – accept yourself even if you're not at your desired weight. Buddhist philosophy tells us when we want what we don't have, we will never be happy. When we begin to appreciate and love what we do have, we'll live in peace with ourselves and with others.

3. Be Mindful of How You Speak to Yourself

If we become aware of what we're telling ourselves, we usually discover we're being disrespected. Most of us don't allow others to speak rudely to us, but somehow we don't blink when we do it to ourselves – mostly because we think we're fat or we eat too much. We need a constant push to make sure we don't keep being undisciplined, right? And then we'll become thin. Sound familiar? Consider creating a self-talk journal for one week. When you find yourself feeling angry, frustrated, sad, or any other challenging emotion, write out your internal dialogue. Like, "I'm so damn frustrated because I ate that stupid piece of carrot cake. I know I'm not supposed to have that! Idiot! I'll never lose weight, and I'll never find the right guy."

You may be shocked by the messages you're sending yourself. But hang on, tiger, because once you start jotting down some of that noise in your brain, you'll have the story – the script – right in front of you. You'll see in black and white how you talk to yourself. Read the script. Ask yourself if it's true. Brace yourself because you may hear a "NO!" And now you can empower yourself and change your life.

Change the script. Using the example above, your rewrite might sound something like this. "I'm fine. I'm good. I'm filled with grace. I'm allowed to have a piece of cake. I was hungry and I wasn't bingeing. When I allow myself to have moderate amounts of the food I love, I no longer want to binge. I'm happy. I love my life. I love myself." You get the idea, the idea being that you're great. The opposite cannot be true.

Cognitive therapy is based on the findings that as you become aware of your scripts and counter them with true, rational thoughts, you'll be able to change your automatic, programmed thinking. And won't that be a refreshing change?

If you get stuck on how to alter those negative thoughts, feel free to ask a friend or therapist, or find a book on how to change your thoughts. One oldie but goodie is *Feeling Good: The New Mood Therapy* by David Burns.

4. Replace False Feelings of Being in Control with Ways to Actually Become Empowered

The serenity prayer always works for us.

God, grant me the serenity to accept the things I cannot change,
the courage to change the things I can,
and the wisdom to know the difference.

How often do you allow the actions of others to ruin your day? Haven't you heard? You have no control over what anyone else believes or the actions they take. But boy, you can drive yourself crazy worrying about something over which you have absolutely no control. If you often find yourself spinning helplessly out of control, reacting with anger or frustration to others, take a few minutes and say the Serenity Prayer. Write it out. Now, think of everything that's troubling you and write those things. Then, under the prayer make two columns: Title one "What I Can Control," and the other "What I Can't Control." Begin sorting. For the problems listed in the "can control" column, write goals and action plans for what you can do – and then chill out, because you won't be able to do every single one of them in a day. (You perfectionists need to give yourselves time.) And for the problems that reside in the "cannot control" column, guess what? You get to say a prayer and – get a load of this – let those problems go! Do it. It works.

5. Stop Weighing Your Self-esteem and Stop All Body-checking

Do you often find yourself turning to the side before the mirror, only to be disappointed by what you see? Do you typically conclude you're too fat or too big and wish you were a different size? Do you weigh yourself often? Do you go nuts with a tape measure around different parts of your body? Do yourself a favor: throw the damn scale and that tape measure away. Have a bonfire for your tight jeans. The more you body-check and rely on the scale, the more often you set yourself up for disappointment. Besides, the scale is not an accurate measure of your worth.

When you choose friends, do you have them turn around first to make sure their asses are hot enough – or do you love people for who they are? You choose friends for the fun times you have, their warmth, and the way they understand you. Make sure your life is filled with people who are genuine – people who allow you to be genuine, too. In the meantime, avoid the scale. And the next time you pass a mirror, consider the fact that a sexy person may be staring back at you.

6. Avoid Comparing, Competition, and Jealousy

Don't we all want what we can't have? The scarcity principle is found in marketing. When something is scarce (or rare) people are more apt to want it – and then they'll be the only ones to have this amazing, coveted thing. Doesn't having a hot body fit this category? A small percentage of people on the planet actually have that perfect hot bod. The more rare it is, the more people want it. Comparing happens. What happens when you go to gym class one day and find your body fat is tested, with all the numbers and names of people posted on the wall. Or, you look around the gym to see who's hottest and start comparing yourself to them. But what good comes of comparing? Either you feel superior to someone or you feel devalued. Are people with lower body fat, or those who weigh less, better than you in some way? Change your inner dialogue. Go from, "I'm so jealous of that guy because he's more popular and better built than I am," to "I'm happy for that guy – he's good looking and I'm so am I. It's a good thing there are enough dates for us all." Change your thoughts, change your life, change your karma.

7. When You Feel Insecure, Do Some Service

Go outside yourself. See yourself being useful, helpful, and kind. See your body as an instrument, not an ornament. Donate time to a nonprofit organization or your spiritual center. You heal yourself when you serve as a catalyst for healing others. Now you'll see yourself for who you truly are; a loving, caring, competent human being.

And one final thought – this from Laura, a thirty-one-year-old video production instructor and documentary filmmaker, who's struggled with body-hate.

    "Get a friend. And don't get just any friend; get a good friend. Find a friend who loves you and tells you she loves love you no matter what. Find a friend who'll listen to you at all hours of the day, hug you when you cry, care about you when you're sad, and stand up for you when you need it most. Whenever I had a moment of really hating my body, which was how I dealt with most feelings, instead of looking in the mirror obsessively, I turned to a good friend. I didn't necessarily tell her how I was feeling. I would just be around her, do something fun with her, and laugh. Being around another person who enjoyed my company made me start to like myself and see my own self-worth. My friend essentially became my mirror, and reflected a part of myself I liked to see. So whenever you have a moment when you hate your body, don't look in a mirror; find a friend. Look into her eyes, have a good laugh, and get a big hug.**"**

"No comparing. No competition. No jealousy.
Repeat, Repeat, Repeat."

—Our Spiritual Advisor

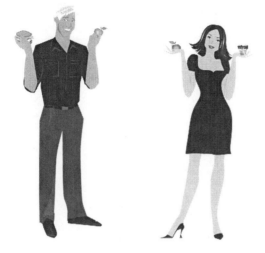

*"I'm so grateful that I don't get on a scale,
because it's never going to be the right number."*
—Kyra Sedgwick, *More Magazine*

Chapter Six
The Scale Is Not Your God

YES. IT'S TRUE, THE SCALE IS NOT YOUR GOD. Do The Ten Commandments say "Thou shalt covet the scale?" No. Nor is it in the American Constitution. Listen to us, and listen clearly, preferably while you're snacking on something yummy, because God knows *we* are doing that right now. DON'T STEP ON A SCALE!

Just don't. Especially if you're already addicted to the damn thing. How do you know if you're obsessed with the scale? If you step on it more than once a week and feel emotionally triggered by the number you see, guess what? You could be an addict – obsessed with body image and size. And, quite possibly, you may be addicted to beating up on yourself.

How many times have you hoped and prayed to the scale God that you could be that *perfect* weight, after spending weeks restricting your food intake, feeling hungry – but feeling oh-so-in control, right? You avoided bad food, remaining hungry while eating good ones. (If only those rice cakes felt substantial, right?) And then, the anticipated day arrived, the day you stepped on the Numbers Beast only to discover ... what? You wanted to see a bigger difference between the number you last spotted between your feet and the one you're currently staring at?

Here's the problem with selecting a weight goal: it's arbitrary. Arbitrary is when you make a choice for no good reason. So shut up about picking numbers out of the sky, imposing them on yourself, and then emotionally flogging yourself when you don't make that weight.

Do you have a current weight goal? How important is it to you? Why did you select that number? Many people choose what they should weigh based on that scale, others use a body fat calculator, others do it by clothes. In fact, we've known people who, for years, didn't go out much because they weren't a certain waist size. Exhausting!

Ask yourself, "How did I select this number?"

The most common answer is, the goal weight equals your lowest weight at one point, probably when you were much younger. Another reason could be it's what a friend or family member weighs. Maybe you picked a weight because it's a nice, round number. Perhaps it's just a bit lower than what you weigh now. Maybe someone else told you what you should weigh. On and on it goes ...

Nancy, a forty-seven-year-old teacher, mother of two, and part-time animal rescuer, shares her story.

66With life so out of control, the one thing I had control over was *the number*; the number on the scale. I needed exercise to get through this rough stretch, but what would be the reward? The number on the scale became my ultimate goal, or maybe obsession is a better word. Trivial really; an analog here, digital there, just a number. I always told myself, "I'm in complete control and can stop any time.

At first, my goal was returning to what I weighed as a senior in high school. I began charting my progress on a graph and recording my workouts on a calendar. Once I reached the first goal, a few more pounds and I'd be in the teens. And so I exercised, and the line on the graph went down. I weighed in every day at the gym wearing approximately the same clothing for consistency. Then, one day, I was cornered by a gym teacher at school who said I was starting to look like a skeleton. "Okay, 115 and I'll stop, No big deal." But when 115 rolled around, that put me only five pounds away from having a zero in my weight, a ZERO! Oh my gosh – how exciting was that? And next – double digits! DOUBLE DIGITS! I was almost there when – sound of door opening – a counselor walked into my life. End of story. Beginning of story. 🙖

How much time energy, blood, sweat, and tears have we put into our weight goals? We know about feeling fat; about trying on ten outfits to find just the right one that doesn't make us look fat; about stepping on the scale and feeling like an utter failure. You're not alone.

Thirty-eight-year-old Michelle, a CPA from Texas got off the merry-go- round after twenty-five years of yo-yo dieting that left her filled with anxiety, shame, and disgust.

🙖I was constantly preoccupied about what my weight had to be, and this left me filled with anxiety and self-hatred. I would weigh myself several times a day. The changes were never great; a pound or a few up and down all the time, but to me, that number was everything. I would be so happy I lost weight, but probably I'd just gone to the bathroom, because how much weight could you actually lose from minute to minute and hour to hour? This went along with trying on half a dozen outfits before going out, and on some nights never finding even one that made me feel okay, so I'd cancel my plans and stay home. On those nights, I'd end up trying to work out, and then got so hungry I'd end up binge-eating on top of it. What a depressing time in my life, and it lasted for so long. Now, it's such a relief to accept my body and myself. My weight doesn't even fluctuate, because my eating and exercise habits are stable. And now my life is stable, too. **99**

Like Nancy and Michelle, you may have selected a mysterious goal weight number. Even more curious is the fact that some people are given a weight by their doctor, a parent, a lover, a health teacher, a sports coach. Hey – and we mean this – we're sorry these people disrespected you. You're responsible for your body. And that means making the right choices about how to feed it, care for it, manage, and maintain it. Your body is yours. Tell everyone else to SHUT UP!

In the meantime, the best way to gain freedom is to avoid the scale. The next step: buy clothes that comfortably fit.

Whoa. Really?

Yeah. What a concept.

You might have to let go of a mind-bending phenomena – wearing tight-fitting clothing because that size once made you feel skinny or fit. Therefore, if you can squeeze into the clothing, you can hang onto the illusion that you're skinny or fit. Meanwhile, your flesh is begging for air.

Enter coauthor Greg. He can't count how many times he yo-yo'd up and down with weight during his teens. He felt chubby growing up and was told he should look thinner – like other guys. In college he lost a ton of weight, but after doing so he became preoccupied with staying at 173 pounds and a size 32 waist. Then everything would be okay. More importantly, that weight and size meant he was thin, cool, good-looking, and accepted. Naturally he gained weight back, but found himself still trying to stuff his body into size 32 jeans that didn't fit. Do you know what happened? He always felt fat.

Stop wearing clothes that are too small for you. This only promotes the inane notion that you're too fat and therefore – what's this? Not beautiful because you're too fat.

Enough!

We've said it before, and we'll repeat it again, because you're worth it and we like you. The more you follow your hunger and fullness cues, the better off you'll be. Do that, along with exercise you love, and you're body will morph into the size it naturally wants to be. Yes, the size it naturally wants to be. Follow those cues and your body will naturally do the rest.

Here's our stellar idea. Instead of stepping on the scale, head to the mirror. In fact, Greg tells the spin students he teaches to go to the mirror every morning and say, "Damn. That is one awesome person staring back at me!" Do it. We also know many people who, on their return from dieting hell, wrote little affirmations and messages to themselves and posted these everywhere they could think of. Can you imagine a mirror covered in positive affirmations? You can't even see the love handles, because for a little while that section of the mirror is populated by sporty notes that say, "I love you!" or "Your body is an amazing gift from God." Maybe you use the car to drive and get binge food. Well, line your car with Post-its that say, "Be careful where you're going right now." Or, "I'm a great person who can achieve my goals."

Try it. And mean it. Because, think about this: how could the opposite be true? It can't. Any personal equation where the sum equals *I am not good enough* is false. Period. End of story. Don't even try arguing with us, because we'll point back to the mirror and remind you how fabulous you are.

Now, where'd we leave those tasty cupcakes?

REALITY CHECKS

Myth: The scale is my friend.

Reality: *No way. It's a scale – an object.* And think about this concept. You're not its friend unless it shows what you want to see.

Myth: Scales accurately capture the state of my health and well-being.

Reality: *They don't. Scales measure body weight.* Period. Your body weight is made up of the water your body is carrying at any given time, PLUS all your muscles and fat – hello, some fat is necessary – and much more (bones, ligaments, blood, etc. Hell, even our brains weigh seven pounds.) The scale does not accurately access a person's true health or self-worth.

Myth: If the number on the scale is bigger than I think it should be, then I'm overweight. (Read: Fat.)

Reality: *Not necessarily. Muscles weigh more than fat.* If you work out and gain muscle mass, you may actually gain weight, but look slimmer and fitter, and even improve your health. For weighing addicts, if you weigh yourself daily or even more frequently, think about what you're actually weighing. Ask yourself, "If I check my weight at 2 p.m. and then try again at 4 p.m. what am I accurately measuring?" Can a person's body mass change in two hours? Nope. Frequent weighers wind up measuring fluid shifts. For people with food and weight concerns, their days can be filled by such shifts – from having a flat stomach, putting on tight jeans and feeling thin (a.k.a. dehydration) to feeling fat, bloated, having trouble getting on rings, and having that tummy stick out. These hourly or daily shifts are not changes in flesh. They're a measurement of body fluid shifts, exacerbated by food restriction, purging and other unhealthy weight-control behaviors, such as taking laxatives, water pills, or diet pills. These methods don't make any difference in your weight, but they do get you caught up in measuring minute changes in water shift throughout the day.

If you still don't believe us, check this for yourself. Weigh a brand new sponge. Let's say it weighs an ounce. Now soak the sponge in water. Maybe it suddenly weighs five ounces. Did the mass of the sponge change? Of course not. This is a good analogy for weighing yourself frequently. You'll only capture – and overreact to – water shifts. If you can relate to this, recognize that you're measuring nothing; you're chasing your tail in a circle. Seek the help of a counselor or eating-body disorder professional as soon as possible. But first – chuck that damn scale.

Myth: "If my jeans are too tight, I must be too fat."
Reality: *Honey, it's not you – it's the damn jeans.* Now, shut up and buy some new ones.

Myth: I will spend a lifetime fighting my natural body size/weight.
Reality: *You don't live in a boxing ring, baby.* Put down the gloves. Quit beating yourself up. Besides, how well has all that fighting worked for you so far?

Myth: I could always be more beautiful if I was thinner.
Reality: *Shut up and go eat something.* Every person is beautiful in every size. Yeah, it's true. We will always be beautiful if we're loving and grateful in our lives.

Teen Myth: I need to weigh what I weighed last year.
Reality: *The SBM (Skinny Bitches Mindset)* leaves no room to live abundantly. Gaining forty to fifty pounds between

the ages of ten and sixteen is normal. In the book *Teaching Body Confidence,* the author notes we gain approximately 20 percent of our adult height and 50 percent of adult weight between the ages of eleven and nineteen. Each of us grows at a different rate, so it's important not to compare ourselves to other people. Easy to say, but again, we've already discussed how most of us have the tenacity and drive to restrict eating. Instead, let your body evolve. Young people often gain weight around the midsection before they grow taller. Their bodies need this extra weight to increase in height. Childhood and teen years are awkward times for the body. Please be kind to yourself and accept the fact that your body may need to carry extra weight at times. In the meantime, have the courage to follow your hunger and fullness cues. It'll all work out, in time.

Adult Myth: If 40 is the new 30, and 60 is the new 40, then I really should make sure my body doesn't change at all as I age.

Reality: *Shut up, and let it go.* Now you're worrying about age? Let's put it this way: Celebs who can afford a personal trainer, a personal chef, a live-in nanny and housekeeper, and all the plastic surgery and liposuction money can buy—even *they* get caught by tabloid photographers who can't wait to show off the cellulite, the bed head, the bloated tummy, the bags under their eyes and, perhaps, "recovering" from too much weight loss after filming something "important." Face it, we need to accept some normal weight gain and weight redistribution over the years. Just because you don't look perfect, doesn't mean you aren't gorgeous or acceptable. Most important is how you *feel*. Great, we hope, because that good feeling creates a beauty radiating from deep within; the type of beauty people really admire.

What to do with your *Tight-Fitting* clothes.

- Give them to charity.
- Turn old jeans into an art project with a set of markers, a sewing machine, and some good friends. You can sew those old jeans into a purse or bag. And look for stores, like the GAP, that take old and used jeans and send them off to be recycled and used as insulation in new buildings. (Yeah, giving up that tight pair of jeans just 'cuz it makes you feel skinny is actually eco-friendly.)
- Think of a person who has an upcoming job interview and could use your old suit.

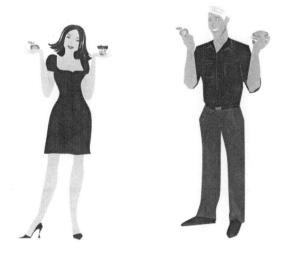

*"Our personality and its defenses, one of which is
our emotionally charged relationship to food,
are a direct link to our spirituality. They
are the bread crumbs leading us home."*

—Geneen Roth,
Woman, Food, and God

Chapter Seven
*Who's Managing Your Food—
You or Your Emotions?*

WOULDN'T LIFE BE GREAT IF WE COULD FEEL what we feel and not have to avoid it? Wouldn't it be awesome if we didn't *have to* make food an emotional bandage to help us cope with all the things we believe we can't handle?

Breakups: "Hello, lovely pint of Ben & Jerry's!"

Work issues: "Come to momma, super-sized bag of Oreos!"

Money woes: "Sure, I'll eat *your* order of fries, too!"

Who among us lovely humans hasn't, at one time or another, eaten in response to all kinds of stimuli other than basic hunger? Often we become stressed about something, and suddenly we've consumed several plates of leftover mac 'n' cheese. Or, we're angry with someone and find ourselves gobbling twice the amount of a typical dinner serving. (Greg used to easily polish off an entire bag of Doritos in one sitting only to later realize that — *what's this?* — he had waves of confusion or loneliness that he didn't know how to deal with.)

It happens.

Then there's the flipside. We're emotionally triggered by something and put off eating like compliant skinny bitches, so by the time we do eat we're so damn hungry we can't make rational choices about food. (Much like when you can't control your breathing after having a plastic bag over your head).

When we ignore our feelings, they build up and have a way of coming back with a vengeance. Worse, we form addictive behaviors when we don't actually deal with core issues that run deep – like way down there, folks. For a great many of us, these behaviors show up in our relationship with food.

Can't speak up to your boss? Make that a twelve-inch sub with extra cheese for lunch.

Having intimacy issues in the bedroom? Nuke some pizza rolls in the microwave.

Unable to say No to a bully? Grab three cupcakes.

This works in reverse, too. Afraid of your upcoming job interview? Suddenly you're not in the mood for lunch. Got yelled at by your dad? The healthy snack goes out the window. Saying yes or no to food in response to emotions is common.

Good news: You're not alone.

Julie, a twenty-one-year-old college student recovering from anorexia and bulimia nervosa, proves this.

> **"**Lately I've been able to look outside of the food. For so long, I tried to control food when I couldn't control other aspects of my life. I now realize that instead of controlling the food, it's controlling me. I've given food that much power – letting it consume my every thought and influence my every

action. But if it's not about the food, what is it about? That's where the answer lies. Sometimes life seems easier if I focus on food rather than actually face what I'm avoiding in the first place. **"**

If there's one habit we need to form, it's opening ourselves to feelings and being willing to effectively deal with them. This process begins when you ask yourself a simple question: **Who's managing my food – me or my emotions?**

Feel free to ask this every time you're about to bite (or refuse to bite) into a culinary wonder, especially if you've had issues around food and self-esteem. This is the single most important question you can ask yourself.

The next question is: What am I feeling?

Ouch.

Sometimes that's too complicated to figure out, right? How do we ever know for sure what we're feeling? At any given time we might be zipping along on our emotional roller coaster, experiencing a gaggle of emotions: fear, doubt, anger, *fear*, excitement, joy, happiness, *fear*, grief, sadness, depression, *fear*, hope, love, lust, *fear*, passion, confusion, hope, FEAR!

Fear much?

Listen, the best brain candy we can give you is permission to ask yourself these two questions:

Who's managing my food – me or my emotions?

And ... What am I feeling?

"All right," you say. "I've asked myself both questions. I realize my emotions are managing my food at the moment, and that right now I'm feeling some fear. What's next?"

Good question. Now what?

Now, the fun begins. Yeah ... fun. It's the new F-Word. Try it on for size. This is much more effective than anything SBMers are doing, which is telling you to be skinny.

Now, you get to understand yourself on a deeper level. Now, you get to see things about yourself you may have never known. Now, you get to heal.

Trust us, this may not taste good going down – who likes to feel stuff that doesn't feel good, right? But the end result is downright satisfying. Why? Because you'll feel the emotion, hopefully integrate it, and move on – as you learn something. Consider dealing with seemingly challenging emotions as if you're passing spiritual gas, folks. (What a relief, right?) And in the end, let's face it, we all have to digest whatever the heck is happening to us inside – literally and figuratively.

At first you may not be accustomed to feeling bad if you aren't numbing your feelings through eating, or self-starving. Numbing? You may not realize how you shove feelings away through food, lack of food, or compulsive exercise. Take note of an excerpt of a poem entitled "Numb" from twenty-four-year-old Kim.

> I like to numb out, using food as a drug,
> curled up in my bed, all comfy and snug.
> No emotions to burn a hole in my heart,
> to remind me that I am not pretty or smart.
>
> No reason or passion, my life is a mess.
> Why feel if it hurts? So empty, depressed.
> Yet, being numb blocks the positive, too,
> joy, peace and love, cannot get through.
>
> My life is a blur, from one binge to the next
> and now I need more, for equal effects.
> It's harsh and progressive; it is a disease,
> though it creates the illusion of comfort and ease.
>
> But nothing is easy when I have to see
> that the mirror's reflection is actually me.

You can sense the depression Kim feels and the role food played in numbing her feelings. Sorting out feelings will help you move away from feeling numb. Then, as Kim points out, you get to experience not only the bad feelings, but the good ones as well.

NOW WHAT? BEHOLD: THE FOOD LOG

Don't roll your eyes. Chances are you, like many others who fell into the SBM trap, had enough energy to restrict food or even binge. Then guess what? Use that same energy and willpower to do something positive – like the simple task of creating a food log. Don't fret. This will be downright illuminating. And don't tell us you can't do it. We know you. We know you can.

The lowdown: Find a notepad or notebook and use it as a guide to make you more aware of what, if any, emotions are attached to some of your food choices during a week's time. Be sure to include emotions during the times you restricted food, since this is a blind spot for many people. The log will make it clear whether boredom, loneliness, or other emotions were part of non-hunger eating. And you know what emotions we're talking about: anger, fear, sadness, depression, nervousness, intimacy issues, cravings for nurturing or love, exhaustion, and fear, fear, fear.

The task? To untangle feelings attached to food. Use this log for several weeks, ideally one month. Write down what you eat and begin connecting the emotions you feel whenever you feed yourself, or choose not to eat by restricting food. Have fun with this. Play detective. For each entry, rate your hunger and fullness levels from 0 to 10.

For example, perhaps you ate twenty cookies or four bowls of cereal when your hunger level was four. What's up with that? Maybe one day you ate an entire bag of tortilla chips when your hunger level was six or seven. Did you have other food choices at the time? Write it all down in the log. What you feel when you begin consuming these kinds of food matters, especially if the emotions are strong.

By recording what you eat and then analyzing the results, you'll soon begin to see the role food plays in your life and decide if there's anything you want to change. Begin to notice similar emotions surfacing. If you find you're often sad, depressed, or anxious when you eat, it's important to explore why this is so. What's underneath all emotion?

Why are you sad?

Why are you depressed?

Why are you anxious?

Ask yourself. No, really – ask yourself these questions. If you don't, who will? Most importantly, it's vital you understand those emotions don't have to be avoided; that you don't *have* to use food to avoid feeling them.

Yes, you, oh marvelous creature that you are, can *feel* and *deal* in a healthy way. You can...

Know what you feel, and why.

Talk to trusted loved ones about problems.

Solve problems effectively.

Suppose you've done this amazing thing – created a food log. You're recording things and taking action. Then, let's say two weeks into the project you take a close look at what you've written. You notice a number of times you ate out of boredom rather than hunger. That boredom turned up many times in the food log. This is an awesome epiphany. This tells us you need to plan fun things to do –and execute those things. So, grab that notepad again. Yes, living is a verb, so taking action is necessary, folks! Make a list of things you love to do, or used to love to do, and several things you'd love to try. Be honest and creative. Include indoor and outdoor activities. Get the materials you need for the items on your list, whether it be hiking shoes, paintbrushes, beading equipment, or whatever. You get the picture. Now you're ready. You may find you need a friend to be with you if you're breaking engrained patterns. Be specific about what you're going to try, and then put it on your schedule; make a few play dates with yourself and others.

Suppose, after some time, you notice that when you aren't eating out of hunger, you're eating out of fear.

Digging deeper, you sense a great deal of fear, perhaps more than you realized. Maybe a counselor or therapist could work with you on unraveling these feelings. While working with a therapist you come to understand the fear is linked to trauma from the past.

We often feel our traumas don't matter. But that's a defense against painful feelings. You tell yourself, "Oh, my trauma isn't big enough, so good, I don't have to go in and deal with it!" But we all tend to carry around unacknowledged trauma, such as being teased – that's a biggie. Other traumas include abandonment, rejection, physical, verbal, or sexual abuse, and even unresolved grief over the loss of a loved one.

One helpful way to see what traumas may be hiding in your psyche is to create a timeline. For each of your years, go back and review significant events (positive or negative) and then check to see if you developed any symptoms with eating based on mood or behaviors around those times. This is all part of connecting the dots to overcome unhealthy eating patterns.

Traumatic events can be challenging for the brain to process. By *process*, we mean make sense of, learn from, and let go of. Some people who experience trauma learn from them. For others, the ability to fully understand what happened to them, psychologically and emotionally, isn't that simple. Sometimes we experience disconnection when it comes to healing and integrating things that happen to us. For example, if the trauma is sexual assault, it's common to learn something erroneous about yourself, your body, or the world.

As a result, an inner dialogue was created to reinforce a belief that isn't grounded in truth. The dialogue might sound like this. "I need to be too thin or too big to be unattractive. That will protect me from being assaulted." Or, "I must be really dumb if I let that happen, so I'll hide away from people to protect myself."

As you can see, these inner conversations don't protect you from something like assault. Assault happens to males and females of all ages, shapes, and sizes. But if we assume it has something to do with our looks, then we feel the need to gain control and protect ourselves. We then generate a series of actions that manifest around food, such as overeating, restricting eating, and the like.

The good news is, many steps can help you work through trauma, from dialoguing about it with trusted friends to counseling. (Hell, we should all get a therapy trust fund when we're born, so we can dip into it during challenging moments of our lives). One way to work through trauma, is to actually write out the story of what happened: Write what we learned about it. Write about our feelings surrounding it. A great deal of this learning is unconscious, so while looking at behavior patterns and eating patterns is a great time to make these connections.

Are you affected by trauma? Note the following common trauma symptoms, according to the research of renowned trauma specialist John Briere.

- trouble falling asleep
- restless sleep
- nightmares
- stomach problems
- headaches
- sadness
- loneliness/isolation
- uncontrollable crying
- guilt and/or shame
- respiratory issues
- desire to physically hurt yourself or others
- being under or overly sexual/having sexual problems
- fear of women or men
- memory problems
- feeling that things are "unreal"/"spacing out" (going away in your mind)
- flashbacks (sudden, vivid, distracting memories)
- anger, irritability or anxiety

Do any of these apply to you? Have you experienced one or more symptoms on an ongoing basis? If you answered yes, that's good. Why? Because you've noticed. Now you can take action. You can love yourself. You can consider therapy and heal. We talked about counseling and therapy before, so here's a tip on finding a therapist. Trust your instincts. You're a smart cookie (no pun intended). You'll know who you can feel safe with as you work through deeper issues – issues that a big bag of chips or skipping breakfast may have helped you mask. Above all, know that exploring these deeper issues is no piece of cake. (Sorry, we're trying to lighten things up.) So many of us have been trained to believe we can't deal with certain feelings or deep issues. But that's exactly what we're here to do on this planet – embrace them. We won't use the onion metaphor, but think of it like this. You're a cupcake and the more you explore your inner world, try to understand who you are, what motivates you, and more, it's like peeling away a portion of that sticky paper cupcake holder.

Okay, that one bites. So let's move on...

Sometimes it isn't easy to know what you're feeling at the time you feel it. Use this little cheat-sheet any time you get emotionally stuck: depressed, bored, sad, lonely, rejected, isolated, celebrating, happy, connected, scared, fearful, avoidant, unmotivated, angry, enraged, unwanted, hopeless, helpless mistrustful, blessed, grateful, loved, affectionate, motivated, in pain, overwhelmed.
Just breathe!
You're in there somewhere and you'll discover new emotional patterns, or revisit old ones. The good news? You're discovering more of yourself.

GOOD AND BAD REDUX

When you begin recording feelings in your food logs, you may notice an interesting array of emotions, especially if you're struggling with a mental list of *good* and *bad* foods. Let's take one of our favorites: Cheetos. If you love the taste of Cheetos but don't often let yourself have them, guess who's going to be in the kitchen (or at the store) calling your name? Cheetos. The Cheetos will say, "Hi, old friend. Remember me? It's been so long since you've had me! I've missed you. And I know you missed me. Just me and you! Just one night!"

You don't have to go through a love/hate battle with Cheetos, or any other yummy food or treat banned by your inner critic and the SBMers. If you want to stop bingeing, consider eating the feared foods in moderation. That way, they'll have no power over you. If you can eat Cheetos anytime you like, then you won't be so anxious when you do. You'll be able to eat them with little conflict or emotion and have the self-control you need to eat without bingeing. This way, your food log can help you embrace foods you once feared.

Your fear of certain foods probably began back in childhood.

"Put down those cookies – don't eat that! You're getting fat!

"Why can't you look like other kids who are thin!"

"No, you can't have cake, it's not healthy for you."

Perhaps you heard words like these while you were growing up. Or maybe when you began to run track you had a coach who constantly harped on what to eat. Think back on the messages you received about eating, and the history of your personal battle with food.

For many of us, patterns of turning to, or away from, food for solace or escape began back in childhood. As kids we often couldn't control whether we were understood or heard. Food was the only thing over which some of us felt we had any control, and often we were right. Especially at risk are kids who have rigid food rules imposed upon them; kids rarely allowed to consume the appetizing foods we all crave. Those children, in particular, are likely to have more issues/conflicts with food, and crave those forbidden cookies more often. An eight-year-old struggling through a challenging time wouldn't realize her cravings for bowls of cereal have something to do with the brain turning the carbohydrates found in cereal into serotonin, a natural anti-depressant that can ease her discomfort. She might notice feeling a little comfort and relief. But notice she isn't solving the underlying issues, but instead developing unhealthy patterns that confuse eating with emotions.

We can gain many insights by looking back on childhood and at children, as twenty-five-year-old Erin, a life coach who's been in recovery from an eating disorder for four years, points out...

66 We hear the phrase *emotional eating* all the time on talk shows and in news segments, and they always say emotional eating is a bad thing. What's not discussed is that eating IS emotional, because most food has emotion tied to it in some way. I like the term Emotional Eating. Taste and smell are two of our strongest senses, and eating something or smelling something cooking that has a memory tied to it - good or bad - can transport you decades back in time. Eating and cooking and exercise should be enjoyable emotional experiences. We need to recognize that it's harmful when we use food and exercise to try and control our emotions.

Actually, we can learn a lot about how to eat and exercise from children. They don't always eat when they're hungry and stop when they're full, and they haven't had their bodies' natural instincts replaced with our thoughts on good/bad foods. They don't condemn themselves to the gym multiple times a week. That's an example we should all follow. Next time you go to an outdoor function, watch the kids. They're playing most of the time and also tasting most of the food. They're on the swings with pieces of candy hanging out of their mouths. It's not just the food that makes them happy, it's the experience as a whole - equal parts of food and activity. Children have the art of balance mastered without even knowing it. One of the most important things I learned was to put down the self-help books and start following the example of those who didn't know they were setting one. Kids understand eating is emotional, because they haven't been taught otherwise. We should follow their example. I've never known a professional who lived more in the moment than kids. **"**

In the journey of moving beyond the good/bad foods paradigm, we should watch out for false alarms. Sometimes we take a normal portion size of food – a dessert, a snack, a bowl of cereal – then allow food rules to make us anxious. We need to understand this is considered normal eating. If you have a serving of cookies, write that in your food log and realize it's normal and isn't going to make you gain three hundred pounds. But if you find yourself eating something like twenty cookies, then you should delve into the questions. What are you feeling? You may find you typically binge during the evenings. You may have the television on. You may be procrastinating on something you should be doing. You may eat right out of the box of food instead of taking the effort to take the correct serving size. All these observations will help you break out of long-standing patterns. Look at yourself with loving eyes. Know you're a good person. You turned to food innocently. Most importantly, know you're getting ready to move on to new adventures with food; you're ready for food to take its rightful place in your life, so it doesn't overcome what's truly important to you.

Remember these two questions:

Who's managing my food – me or my emotions?

What am I feeling?

You do not have to fear food.
You have to *manage* food.

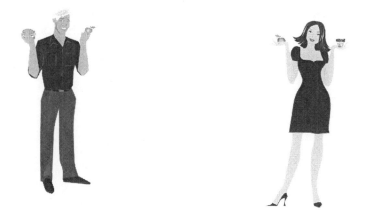

"I've never confessed it [bulimia] before. Out of shame, I suppose, or embarrassment—or just because it's such a strange thing for someone like me to confess to. People normally associate it with young women—anorexic girls, models trying to keep their weight down, or women in stressful situations, like Princess Diana."

—John Prescott,
former Deputy Prime Minister, UK

Chapter Eight
Shut Up, About Excluding Guys

KENNY LOVED SIXTH GRADE. He excelled at his favorite subjects, math and science, discovered he was actually more alert in history class than most of his friends, and he was considering joining the band. But halfway into the first quarter, his body began to change. He gained weight around his mid-section and began feeling awkward about his height, wanting to be taller like some of the other guys. A few weeks before Thanksgiving break he sat down for lunch in the school cafeteria and overheard somebody at the table behind him comment, "Oh, there's that fat kid!" It happened two more times in less than a week.

Kenny didn't eat lunch in the cafeteria for the rest of the year. By spring he was often skipping the meal entirely, only to later binge on cheese sandwiches, chips, or pizza rolls when he got home from school in the afternoon. One day his mother caught him and scolded him for it. "Why can't you be thin like the other boys?"

Kenny felt as if he'd been kicked in the stomach. From that point on, he binged in a special, secluded space – the basement.

Juan came out as a gay man when he was twenty. It was beyond liberating. His teen years were filled with angst, many questions, and what seemed like a never-ending ride on the self-esteem merry-go-around. Juan thought after coming out he'd finally feel free to be himself. But not long after a move to a large metropolitan city, he found himself feeling insecure about his appearance. It began whenever he walked through the town's gay neighborhood. There, he was surrounded by images of perfectly toned men, most sporting bodies fine-tuned in the gym – with defined muscles and tight-fitting clothing that revealed their physiques. Suddenly, Juan felt the urge to work out more. His new friends were totally fit, after all, and they only wore the coolest clothes that showed off their hot bods. Besides, Juan reasoned, there was nothing wrong with being healthy. Why not workout?

Juan frequented the gym nearly every day during the next two months. He took three spin classes a week, two other aerobics classes, plus body sculpting classes, and couldn't wait for the next workout. A bunch of guys his age were wearing skinny designer jeans and he thought, "I want to fit into those." So he did everything he could to do just that. Sometimes, he'd skip meals in lieu of protein shakes or protein bars. It worked. Juan was thin and felt he looked great in size 28 jeans. But he was always tired. He felt sluggish and didn't have any energy until noon, after the java drinks he consumed kicked in. One day somebody told he needed to bulk up; work out with a trainer. Juan followed their advice and for the next six weeks worked hard at adding muscle mass, but the problem Juan soon discovered: his naturally lanky body wouldn't bulk up. Did he want to look like the other guys with their big chests and biceps, or did he want to still fit into skinny jeans? He couldn't decide.

Juan felt more confused about himself and his relationship to his body than before coming out.

Twenty-four-year-old Joey shares this story about his eating disorder.

> **"** I first got it when I was sixteen or seventeen years old. I played football and baseball in high school and this started in the winter between the two seasons. I was heavy as a young person. My mom was overweight, and I saw how painful it was for her. I got heavier in eighth grade, then in high school I thinned out as I grew. But I still hated myself and saw myself as a heavy person.
>
> I was good at baseball and I wanted to play in college. I would "eat healthy" and exercise to make up for anything I ate. I see now I was restricting and over-exercising, and I was way too hungry. One day while running, I was so nauseous from the heat and not eating that I threw up. That's when it hit me to purge. This was the only way I could run a little bit less, and it soon became the only way I felt comfortable eating at all. I was able to play college baseball, but with my eating disorder I couldn't enjoy it. I became an alcoholic because I either couldn't look at myself or hated what I saw. Being drunk allowed me to stop the self-hatred for a little while because I didn't have to think about it. **"**
>
> (Thankfully, Joey has been in recovery from alcoholism and the eating disorder for over one full year.)

Chances are, you may know someone like Kenny, Juan, or Joey. If you do, it's high time to tell the skinny bitches out there who insist we look a certain way, "Shut up, about excluding guys!"

Welcome to the new reality. Women and young girls aren't the only humans pressured to look thin or different. But rarely do we hear discussions about the male side of the equation. The majority of men in America are pressured to lose weight, be thinner, and also "bulk up" and be muscular.

Wait – what are they supposed to do again? Get thinner if they're *fat* but then gain more weight to bulk up? Lose weight, but pack on the muscles? Do you see the insanity here? You can't get real thin and pack on a bunch of muscles at the same time. Muscles, remember, weigh more than fat, so if you're aiming to gain muscle mass, guess what? You're going to carry that weight around, which will make men and young males heavier than they may think they need to be.

Men and boys who are overweight now or have been in the past are susceptible to life-long, deep, and intense body dissatisfaction and low self-esteem – not to mention eating problems. Once you're overweight and you get feedback saying you should be thinner – along with the negative consequences related to that, like feeling unattractive and left out – the chances run high of having a body image disorder.

A man can feel unattractive, unacceptable, and spend a great deal of time looking in the mirror to see if his stomach is getting smaller, or bigger. When men can't fit into the clothes they want to wear – skinny and sexy clothes – they often come down hard on themselves. Worse, it's not cool to worry about your body if you're a guy, so many men are unable to talk about the problem and ask for support.

Who or what is responsible for perpetuating these false truths? We targeted five main culprits, but we could add plenty more.

1. Barbie

2. Male Sexism

3. Media images

4. Specific media images and issues in gay male culture

5. Pressure from participating in sports.

BARBIE

Come on. We all want to say it. **Shut Up, Skinny Bitch!**
Please! If there's a worse role model for young girls, come out,

come out, wherever you are. But here's the thing: Barbie gets all the attention when it comes to perpetuating the unrealistic image young girls and women are supposed to copy. But who knew she had more marketing *cajones* than – drum roll, please – G.I. Joe? When it comes to talking about warped images, G.I. Joe isn't even mentioned. Yet, millions of young boys get the doll, play war, and marvel at Joe's hulking biceps and shoulders. They're conditioned to think that if and when they grow up to look like Joe, wow – won't life be awesome? Won't they be great? And only then will they look right for our society.

But, like skinny bitchin' Barbie, isn't G.I. Joe's pumped-up physique unrealistic? Isn't he as poor a role model for boys as Babs is for the estrogen set?

You bet.

And there are plenty of drawn characters in popular video games, with bodies so perfect, they could never exist in real life. Talk about comparing yourself and coming up short.

Guys are brainwashed at young ages to look tough and be tough. Which brings us to...

MALE SEXISM

Pass the Kleenex. Yes, as in the tissues. As in ... please pass some Kleenex to the boys and let the fellas cry. The fact that society frowns upon this is a form of sexism.

Face it, we consistently overlook the insecurities and emotional concerns of males. Think about it. Is there enough compassion for the concerns of young guys? We say, No.

Males are human, too. They have needs. Why should their need to cry be any less significant than females, who are allowed and even expected to cry? For some reason, men crying and expressing real emotion is still considered weak. Sure, we've made a few strides in shifting this belief, but overall, American society wants men to be macho, tough, hunky, handsome and, occasionally, slightly metrosexual, just to keep everybody guessing.

We need to give boys permission to cry. But, by the age of four, males learn crying is frowned upon if they want to be accepted by their peers and society in general. Therefore, one of the most significant ways human beings take care of their emotions (crying) is suddenly off limits.

Imagine being told you can no longer express the most natural of human emotions. You must suppress it to fit in.

The emotional ripple of these attitudes leads us to believe men have a greater need to use eating and/or restricting food, exercise, and other indirect methods of self-soothing – drugs, alcohol, exercise, gambling – to deal with this lack of emotional expression.

But another nefarious foe lurks out there, and once again, it's...

THE MEDIA

For every picture of a perfect female shoved in your face every day, there's *The Perfect Guy* right beside her. The image usually shows how easy it is to be perfectly pumped up, while not being fat. You'll see these images on billboards, photoshopped in magazine layouts, and on television and in movies. The pressure on guys is immense. For the athlete who wants to look and perform just right, for men who believe they're overweight, for those who've been teased or don't have a great deal of sexual confidence, for those who grow up in families with rampant food and weight concerns: for all these males, we encourage you to realize you're much more than just your body.

You need to be loved for who you are. Not giving yourself permission to feel can hold you back. You're allowed to heal and come back from these issues, just as women do.

SPECIFIC MEDIA IMAGES CATERING TO GAY MALE CULTURE

Gay males often feel heavy pressure to fit a specific look. You'll see that look by browsing the ads in LGBT magazines like "Out," "Genre," or even online at Advocate.com. There, you'll encounter countless images of scantily-clad young lads, buffed hunks, and lean "twinks." "Look male!" the images cry. "Be buff and tone," they urge. "Be a strong man, like this guy!" they scream.

Gay culture has a severe body-centered focus. The expectations for physical appearance are extremely high – much like what we've already noted about women feeling pressured to maintain an ideal body image. And, to add salt into an already open wound, over the last decade those images are loaded with yet another demand: Look young!

So, not only are gay males supposed to be fit; handsome; have a nice, tight ass; big pecs; perfect shoulders; big biceps—exhausted yet? – fit perfectly into tight jeans; smell good on a Saturday night; and give off the best sensual vibe; they're also pressured to look young.

And, if you're over thirty? Next!

Many gay men spend a significant part of their lives trying to be themselves and be accepted, yet when they do come out, they're inundated with media messages that insist, in essence, "You're not good enough, please change!" Talk about irony. That's the exact message they spent most of their lives fighting against.

Pass the celery sticks, right? Well, no. Please pack on the muscles, bro!

Oh, all these mixed messages! But please don't cry about it. Kidding aside, most males don't cry. Chances are, they'll binge – after restricting their eating, of course.

SPORTS AND THE PRESSURE TO BE A *REAL MAN*

Oh, how we love our athletes. America cherishes its football, basketball, and baseball players. It's hard not to. These are magnificent athletes and role models, after all. We admire their will, determination, and physical stamina. They show us anything is possible and nothing is too good to be true, if you're determined and work hard.

Even though professional sports are entertaining, behind the scenes the pressure is intense. These ideals trickle down to *every man*. Much as G.I. Joe shapes the minds of young boys, today's athletes influence male culture. Yet few of us stop to consider the real psychological effect on average guys – as in forming body image disorders and battling low self-esteem.

No way – guys are strong, right? Body image issues don't cross anybody's mind. But not anymore. One sport in particular leads to body image disorders, binge-eating, dieting, and more: wrestling.

Wrestlers are often pressured to be in a lower weight category, because the thinking goes: you'll be more likely to win matches. This heightened weight awareness is a tremendous risk factor for food-related issues. Imagine the overwhelming pressure from coaches and teammates to meet a target weight goal. During weigh-ins, a wrestler over the target weight by even .01 pounds is disqualified from the meet. It's highly competitive. Only one person can wrestle per weight class. College teams, for instance, have ten weight classes; high schools have fourteen, and seventy to eighty kids may be on each team.

All this falls upon a young boy's shoulders. They can't control the rules imposed on athletics, but one thing an athlete *can* control is his body. Wrestlers feel they can control losing weight, cutting fat, and building muscle.

Yes. That pro-weight loss thing goes on in schools, too. Gym teachers and health teachers tell guys to count calories. And how about posting everyone's body fat report on the locker room wall, then giving a day off to the kids who drop a significant amount of fat?

Translation: we're rewarded more for losing weight than for being exactly who we are. Here's a story from Jeff, a twenty-six-year-old teacher who's been in recovery from bulimia for five years.

> "When I was young, we had a lot of stress in my family, and I ate to cope with it. I often overstuffed myself out of stress, and had such a nervous stomach that I was often sick. The family of one of

my best friends constantly compared our weights and bodies. They even put their fingers around our wrists to check who was the thinnest. When I began wrestling, the sport finally sent me fully into an eating disorder. I was surrounded by muscular guys, and I watched the older guys. The message was, "If you want to be great, you need to look like us." The older guys, who were successful and state champs were known to use laxatives and diuretics, make themselves vomit, and work out for hours at the gym. My own problem grew bigger over time. At first, I had my eating disorder only during wrestling season. You have to yo-yo diet because you have to be big and strong, and work out all the time ... and then cut weight for weigh in. If you don't make your weight class, you can't qualify for the meet. This was super competitive, because we had forty people on the team and only ten could start. The pressure was crazy. You had to keep getting bigger and stronger, yet still make your weight. My natural weight was around 150, but my wrestling weight was 133. Some coaches believe cutting down to an extremely low weight makes you a better wrestler. **"**

When the season ended, Jeff says he would be starving.

" I'd balloon up after the season because I could NOT control my eating. I went into the hospital twice at the end of two seasons. I hated myself for the behavior, but I had no way of stopping. I literally lost control. My college coach saved my life. He was the biggest influence in my recovery, because he told me, "No more cutting weight." He changed my wrestling weight to 149, right in my natural weight zone. No more dieting and fighting my own body. And if anyone says you have to cut weight to

wrestle strong, guess what? When I wrestled at 149,
I was able to eat, take care of myself, and be my
strongest. And that's when I became All-American. 🙶

Jeff illuminates how a great many wrestlers struggle with eating
and weight issues. He also reminds us that eating disorders among
high school and college male athletes are more prevalent than people
realize.

🙶Sports and working out can get you totally
focused on body image. Some of the guys would
be in the gym all the time, focusing on their bodies,
and some obviously took steroids.

Affirmations were super helpful for my recovery.
At first, it was hard to believe that by just saying
something you could change your self-perception.
But you have to write it or say something before
you'll ever believe it. By doing so, you can change
your whole paradigm.🙶

PUMP UP ON SOME STATS

Now that we've gobbled up that buffet, let's explore statistics
that clearly illuminate the emotional plight of males.

The *Eat Among Teens* studies (EAT) performed by the Minnesota University School of Public Health surveyed two-thousand
five-hundred teens across five years. Because more than one-
hundred studies were published from this data, we'll direct you to
their website.[5]

The stats tell us a full 30 percent of males are dissatisfied with
their bodies. They feel shame and fear of being unacceptable and
rejected, perhaps because 50 percent believe they should be thinner,
and 50 percent think they should be heavier and more muscular.
Overall, girls hate their bodies and want them to be smaller. But guys

[5] University of Minnesota, School of Public Health. *Project EAT (Eat Among Teens)*:
http://www.sph.umn.edu/epi/research/eat/index.asp

are in a double bind – expected to be simultaneously large, muscular, trim, and slender.

There's more.

- One in eight boys (out of 100,000) between the ages twelve and eighteen, reported using dietary supplements. And who knows what the hell is in those drugs, since most of that industry is unregulated.
- One-third of adolescent males were desperate enough to use unhealthy weight control methods while attempting to lose weight.
- The 6 percent of males who were vegetarian were more likely to be involved in unhealthy weight control behaviors.
- Thirty-two percent of males used skipping meals, diet pills, and smoking more cigarettes to lose or control weight.
- Four percent of males reported taking laxatives, diuretics, vomiting after meals, or fasting.
- About 5.4 percent of males reported steroid use. Steroid use was statistically associated with the following: participation in sports that emphasize weight and shape, disordered eating, substance abuse, parental concern about weight, lower self-esteem, more depressed mood, and suicide attempts.

These guys are trying so hard to do great in sports and be accepted by peers and family. Guys, we love you! Please talk to a friend, a colleague, a school counselor, or someone else you can trust. Find your way back – to you! This particular study stunned many researchers because among other things, it revealed males who were dissatisfied with their bodies actually exercised less over time. This didn't surprise us. These guys were freakin' hungry! The energy needs of teen males are extremely high, and these young men were trying to fit in, be acceptable, listen to their doctor's advice, and avoid teasing and rejection. So they eat less, which leads to lack of energy, diet failure, and binge-eating and decreased activity level to boot.

GAY AND BISEXUAL MEN

In April 2007, the *International Journal of Eating Disorders* reported on a Columbia University's Mailman School of Public Health's study that found gay and bisexual men have a higher risk for developing eating disorders than heterosexual men.

Guess what. Those statistics didn't make the evening news.

Once again, we're here to tell everybody: Shut up, about excluding guys!

The eye-opening study included 516 participants (126 straight men and 390 gay or bisexual men and women). Here's one of the most illuminating stats: At some point, more than 15 percent of gay or bisexual men suffered from anorexia, bulimia, binge-eating disorder, or had certain symptoms of those disorders. A full 5 percent of heterosexual men suffered from those same disorders.

Think about that. We don't often believe males experience this. Perhaps it's time we begin to take notice.

Then there's the stunning documentary film *Do I Look Fat?* by filmmaker Travis Mathews, which beautifully explores eating disorders and body image among gay men. Low self-esteem is the most significant common link among the men featured in the film. This might be, as the film points out, because they were gay or had been overweight, but basically all the guys had been ridiculed for being themselves – and they all used food to deal with tremendous pain. It didn't take long for anorexia and/or bulimia, and other forms of bingeing to enter the picture.

On the Internet site gay.com, writer Marc Breindel commented, "Once a young person internalizes the negative messages repeated by bullies and others, he's vulnerable to self-abuse ... if he's been taught he's responsible for being as 'masculine' as possible, he may become obsessed with looking lean and hard."

The outcome for boys and men – and really for all of us – is the fact that it's toxic to believe we do *not* have a right to feel emotions. This belief spawned a society where most men are not fully dealing with significant issues. In truth, doesn't most information about eating disorders focus on statistics that include only females? One last irony: As you push yourself to have less body fat — you know, so you can be "sexier" — your "hotness" might backfire on you. Persistent low body fat decreases both sperm count and testosterone levels.

Hey guys. We get it. We know you've been left out of the conversation for too long. We want to acknowledge it here. So, follow our lead. You've got balls. Say, "Shut Up, Skinny Bitches!" (Or is it Skinny Bastards?)

Every one in eight boys (out of 100,000), ages twelve to eighteen, reported using dietary supplements.

~Project EAT (Eat Among Teens)

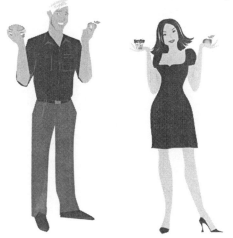

*"I finally know who I am without Ed [an eating disorder]
and I learn more and more about myself every day. I will
never stop learning. Some of the things I have learned:
I am funnier than I thought; I am more intuitive
than I believed. I am more in love with life
than I ever imagined possible."*

—Jenni Schaefer,
Goodbye Ed, Hello Me

Chapter Nine
Invisible to the Eye: Eating Disorders

PATRICK WAS A YOUNG PILOT when he had to make an emergency
landing in a cornfield. The next time he flew, his anxiety level became
so high that he vomited. And this marked the beginning of Patrick's
battle with bulimia nervosa. For sixteen years he faced on ongoing
struggle to keep food down. And even though Patrick recently
overcame bulimia and now maintains a normal, healthy eating
pattern without purging, he noticed that when he stopped purging he
was overwhelmed by something else: suppressed memories of sexual
abuse. Suddenly his mind flooded with images from his past – things
he'd forgotten until he began recovering from the physical part of
his eating disorder: bulimia. Now, Patrick's journey has changed
course. It revolves around healing emotionally from his abuse and
understanding the role symptoms of eating disorders played in his
life.

Rhonda is a sixteen-year-old with a major fear of becoming fat.

Her mother is slightly overweight, and Rhonda physically resembles her mom in some ways. Her dad's subtle disapproval over his wife's weight left a vivid impression on Rhonda. Since eighth grade, Rhonda has been serious about eating and exercise. At first it appeared to be normal dieting, but at some point Rhonda's concerns about weight, coupled with eating restriction, developed into a full-blown obsession. She cared more about avoiding weight gain than anything else.

As a result, she withdrew from her friends, became secretive, and often exhibited anger. Over time, her parents noticed the significant change in Rhonda and naturally became alarmed. They took their daughter to the family doctor, who informed them Rhonda's weight was within the normal range and she was fine. Time passed, and Rhonda's condition grew worse. By the time she was officially diagnosed with eating disorder – NOS, she was confined to a wheel chair in the in-patient eating disorders unit of a hospital, and she had a severely low heart rate. It took two full days of fluid intake and nutritional supplements to increase Rhonda's heart rate to a level of recovery so she could do something as simple as walk safely.

How could Patrick suffer with his illness for all of those years without anyone noticing? How could Rhonda's parents be told she wasn't suffering from an eating disorder?

Eating disorders are serious, deadly, and all too common. Twelve million people in the United States have been diagnosed with anorexia or bulimia nervosa. Another twenty-five million suffer from binge-eating disorder, also known as compulsive overeating. Twenty-five percent of men and 45 percent of women are on a diet on any given day, and 35 percent of normal dieters progress into pathological dieters. Twenty-five percent of them will progress into full eating disorders.

Thanks to society's worship of thinness, many people with eating disorders are misunderstood and misdiagnosed. You can't tell by looking at people if they have a disorder, unless they happen to appear deadly thin. With most of these folks, no one can tell they have an illness.

This is where we lovingly say, "Shut up! and listen to us for a moment."

Be careful what you wish for, dieters, because you might get it. And the prize for being the most compliant, über dieter of all? An eating disorder. That's right. This could be all yours if you...

- insist on stopping yourself from eating when you're hungry,
- give yourself rules on how to eat properly,
- constantly criticize your every move and obsess about eating and body image,
- become super anxious about every food choice you make,
- obsess about every pound, calorie, fat gram, or other numbers you use to measure your self-worth,
- avoid eating, and when you actually do eat, search for food that is perfectly healthy, and then find ways to compensate for what you consumed, and/or
- pick apart your body from head to toe, and beat yourself up about real or imagined flaws.

The American Psychiatric Association classifies people with eating disorders into three main categories. The first two are anorexia nervosa and bulimia nervosa. The third category is comprised of people who don't fit the other categories (like Rhonda) and it's dubbed – the Not Otherwise Specified (NOS) eating disorder. Fifty-two percent of diagnosed eating disorder sufferers fall into the NOS category. Since most eating disorders don't fit the main diagnostic categories, it appears something is off kilter with the classification system. Yes, we're not fans of the current system. This rigid, simplistic classification system places most people who suffer from eating disorders into the confusing NOS category.

Let's take a look at these disorders.

Anorexia nervosa is defined as the intense fear of eating and becoming overweight. It includes an obsession with eating and body weight, along with highly restrictive eating and self-starvation. To meet the stringent criteria for a diagnosis of anorexia, you must weigh below 85 percent of your ideal body weight, and females must miss three or more menstrual periods. The strict requirements needed to meet this diagnosis leave many self-starving people feeling invalidated. And what about guys? They don't get menstrual periods. What if you're only 90 percent below your ideal weight? What if you began at 85 percent below your ideal weight, but then gained weight in recovery? Does that suddenly mean you magically don't have anorexia the minute you're 86 percent of your ideal weight? What if you began dieting at a higher than ideal body weight? You could lose a great deal of weight, which would greatly compromise your health, but you still wouldn't meet the criteria for being anorexic.

This weight-based classification totally misses the true mark of what anorexia is all about: self-starvation, intense fear of eating and weight gain, and a distorted body image. We've met many people who have all the characteristics of anorexia, except for low weight. This is especially important because you don't need to be underweight to experience the deadly health risks spawned by weight loss, starvation, erratic eating, and dehydration.

Bulimia nervosa refers to people who eat large amounts of food and then compensate for eating in some way. Basically, they struggle with an obsessive desire to get rid of calories. Enter purging. This can be done through vomiting food (as Patrick did), compulsively over-exercising, or abusing laxatives, diuretics, or diet pills – all in an effort to reverse the effects of food. But take note, beautiful reader. If you haven't tried these methods of weight control, no need to. They're not effective, and – you guessed it – they don't lead to weight loss. Most people with bulimia nervosa are not underweight. The majority fall into the overweight category.

These categories don't accurately reflect what eating disorders are all about.

Binge-eating disorder, also known as compulsive overeating, is the most common type of eating disorder. But this diagnosis doesn't even get it's own category. Instead it's lumped in the Eating Disorder-NOS dumping ground. People with binge-eating disorder struggle with binge eating – it's similar to bulimia, but without purging. Binge-eaters often restrict fats, carbs, and calories in between binges, setting them up to binge again later. Being a good little dieter feeds right into the problem.

Eating disorder – NOS is an ominous category. Here's where all the misfits end up – those who don't fit any other category. No clear distinction tells us which eating disorders go here, and the diagnosis doesn't offer real validation for people who desperately need it. Examples of those in the NOS category include people who purge, but don't binge; females who haven't missed three consecutive menstrual periods; people who chew and spit out food; and anyone who starves and/or over-exercises but isn't 85 percent below ideal body weight.

RETHINKING THE TERMINOLOGY

The more you learn about eating disorders, the more you realize the above categories are entirely too narrow and naively defined. Because the truth about people with eating disorders, including bulimia nervosa and binge-eating disorder, is that at their core they refer to people who mainly suffer from the behavior and desire to *restrict* food, which is why recovery is so difficult.

Digest this. Most bulimic and binge-eaters want to stop bingeing, but they don't want to stop restricting their food. Take that in, because it's an important distinction and comes down to this: these fine folks don't understand the reason they binge is because their nutritional needs aren't being met throughout the day. In most cases, they're trying to make up for under-eating by overeating, which keeps them locked into a futile cycle of behavior.

Eating disorders shouldn't depend on body weight. Instead, they should be defined by a person's thoughts, behavior, and quality of life.

Beyond that, designating anorexia and bulimia as the only disorders with actual names creates a political and social pecking order within eating disorders. To society at large as well as the medical community, anorexia is the most respectable and significant eating disorder. In many eating disorder programs, people who aren't as thin as those with anorexia feel inferior to them. Many patients have said, "I'm just not thin enough to be here!"

The unspoken worship of thinness leaves onlookers simultaneously in awe of, and critical of, the anorexic. People worry about the anorexic's health, yet at the same time, many admire their strength and determination to say "No" to food in a way others can't. How many times have we heard the quip, "I wish I could have a little bit of anorexia?" We wish you could see the sadness on the face of an anorexic who's heard that statement. Inside, they're thinking, "Wow, you just don't get it, because if you felt like I did for one second, you would never want this."

The current method of classifying eating disorders sets up an elitist system where the thinnest receive all the attention, and it leads people to believe weight is the main issue. People who aren't underweight, which includes about 70 percent of those with eating disorders, are invalidated. They constantly feel confused about their disorder and misunderstood by family and friends, most of whom think it's all about weight. "You don't look like you have an eating disorder," friends and family may say. Too many champion starvers never receive the understanding they need, because we don't acknowledge the depth of their pain.

A person's mindset truly defines an eating disorder – the drive to restrict food combined with a significant reduction in the quality of life. Analyzing eating disorders through a research technique called *factor analysis* illuminates all the underlying issues. Note the five factors that truly define an eating disorder.

1. Strong, Persistent Drive for Thinness

Left unattended, the desire for thinness clouds judgment. For example, the person sets a weight goal to lose five pounds, and then moves to another goal the minute the first is accomplished. In the end, satisfaction is fleeting. The drive for thinness becomes more important than anything else. This drive consumes their lives, isolates them from others, and changes their interest patterns. They feel as if they've lost themselves on a people-pleasing quest for thinness. Over time, they move beyond the people-pleasing mindset. They're working for a new master – an eating disorder they serve and listen to at all times. Unfortunately, they can never please it, and their self-esteem plummets.

2. Preoccupation and Fear of Eating and Being Overweight

How much time each day do you spend asking yourself what you should eat, what to do about something you ate, what not to eat, what your body looks like, what to wear, how fat you are, and other such questions? What do you consider a healthy amount of time to think about this topic? Five percent of your time? Twenty percent? Thirty percent? People with eating disorders spend 70, 80, 90 percent, or more, of their time focused on such thoughts. Many professionals now consider eating disorders to be a type of anxiety disorder related to obsessive compulsive disorder. Imagine how nervous and fearful the person is who questions every single food choice and frets about weight all day long. This is a terribly painful way of life.

3. Body Dissatisfaction

Body dissatisfaction is extremely high for people with eating disorders. Many sufferers are so preoccupied and ashamed of their bodies that they shower with the lights off. Imagine that! For most, the longer they look at a photo of themselves, the more flaws they find. Others can't find any photos of themselves because they've ripped them all up. And then, there's clothing. How long does it take to choose an outfit to wear? Many people are engaged in an all-out war with their bodies and spiral into an emotional whirlpool of self-hatred. What can be sadder?

At sixteen years old, Nina is a future author who loves to read and write. She's in her first year of recovery from an eating disorder.

> ❝I clearly remember the feeling of hatred I held inside of me when I was deep into my eating disorder (ED). My body was never good enough. ED is never satisfied. A tiny sliver of me wanted to be normal again. "You're beautiful!" it screamed. But I wouldn't listen. On many nights I stood in front of my mirror and cried because I was always at war with myself.
>
> "Ewww—Look at all this fat!" and then, "NO—what fat? You're skinny!" I'd fight back.
>
> And then, "You're not good enough. Nobody likes you.
>
> "I was convinced the skinnier I could make myself, the better life would be. People liked the thin, pretty models in the magazines, so they would like me, too, right? I wanted to smash my mirror in frustration, despite the seven years of bad luck. I just wanted to be at peace. But it would never happen. The war kept raging inside me – no matter what I did.❞

4. Perfectionism

People with eating disorders tend to be hard on themselves. They beat themselves up over how they look, what they say, and who they are. Perfectionism promotes feeling like an utter failure. Nothing they ever do is good enough and they fail to give themselves credit for anything. They feel worthless. If someone doesn't like them or is angry at them, if they receive a less than perfect grade – in the mind of someone suffering from an eating disorder, this translates to Utter and Complete Failure. It's all about internal search and destroy. A great deal of this stems from the deep fear that someone will discover they aren't good enough. But on the surface, no one could guess how tortured they are inside. How could we? They constantly try to shield themselves by creating a perfect emotional mask, but inside they're in pain; inside, they're hiding.

Twenty-three-year-old Caitlin, a nursing student, knows perfectionism all too well.

> 66 Perfection was all about self-control for me. In my eating disorder this was one thing I could hang onto that I believed I could control, but in reality, it controlled me. It gave me a sense of safety in a world that seemed so out of control. If I could be perfect, then everything would be okay. The worse the eating disorder became, the higher my standards rose. I could always do better. The bar kept moving higher – always out of reach. Nothing was good enough. With the eating disorder, I had to be skinner, lose that much more weight, and be that much sicker. It got to a point where I couldn't stop. I lost sight of who I was. Being perfect didn't seem so good any more. I was losing everything, and my life was falling apart, crashing down on top of me. But to stop, to give up that control, meant failure in my eyes. It meant I wasn't good enough or strong enough. I was weak and everyone would see it. 99

5. Binge-eating

Binge-eating usually develops in dieters and/or food restrictors because their behavior revolves around fighting a big animal: hunger. Some people may be able to fight off binge-eating, at times, but this is hard work. They continually distract themselves from their hunger or cravings and become increasingly obsessive so they can avoid explosions of massive eating. Many people with eating disorders eat erratically. They alternate between periods of severe restricting and periods when their eating feels out of control.

Let's try to capture the big picture about eating disorders, According to a 1994 study, 82 percent of eating disorder patients who were hospitalized had an additional mental health diagnosis. The top three diagnoses were clinical depression, anxiety disorder, and substance dependence (alcohol or drug dependence).

Eating disorders are complicated. If someone you love has an eating disorder, please try to understand what it would be like to go through life with constant doubt, fear, and uncertainty. These disorders are fear-based. Try to comfort and support your loved one, knowing he or she is afraid.

DEATH THREAT

You can't see or know who's going to die from an eating disorder. According to a 2009 study published in the *American Journal of Psychiatry*, the mortality rates for eating disorders are between 4 and 5 percent. Would you feel comfortable having a disease with a 4 or 5 percent mortality rate? This study indicated people of all weights can die from eating disorders, not just folks who are underweight. In fact, the highest death rates were found in the NOS eating disorder category, followed by bulimia. No, the thinnest aren't the only ones who die from eating disorders.

Many people still don't understand that there isn't a direct correlation between what you eat and what you weigh. People naturally want to believe they can establish complete control over body weight by controlling food intake. Yet, some people who eat restrictively don't lose weight. Over time, they'll probably binge. Many factors other than eating control our weight: hormones, sleep, metabolism, activity level, body fat percentage, and more. And, none of these are an exact science. The more you mistreat your body, the more it fights back. If you starve yourself, your body will retaliate and hang onto any nutrition it can.

This is serious business. The 4 to 5 percent who die from their disorders succumb to medical complications related to the eating disorder. Malnutrition and dehydration can create electrolyte imbalances that can lead to heart attacks. Restricting food, engaging in too much physical activity (especially without proper hydration or in severe heat) and purging via vomiting, diuretics, or laxative abuse – all this puts a person at risk for electrolyte imbalance. Add a heart that's been abused through the same malnutrition problems and the risk increases.

There's also a medical risk in *re-feeding*. A person who's been severely malnourished and begins eating again may experience re-feeding syndrome, whereby the body retains too much water and the ankles swell as the compromised body attempts to incorporate new nutrition. Re-feeding syndrome can occur in all weight groups. Surprisingly, this can even be a concern for bariatric surgery patients, although one would assume they couldn't be malnourished because they're considered obese.

People recovering from any eating disorder need medical care to make certain nutritional rehabilitation is safely carried out.

Malnutrition starves the body, mind, and soul. That's why the leading cause of death among eating disorder sufferers is suicide. We noted earlier that depression, anxiety, substance abuse, and other psychiatric conditions often coexist with eating disorders, which makes this kind of situation more complicated and potentially more dangerous.

Imagine the scenario: you're suffering from an eating disorder, you're confused, you want to fit in. You go on a quest to have that "perfect body" and do everything in your power to look good – please your family, your friends. You do this often, sometimes for years. And you're actions often result in restrictive eating and self-criticism. You just don't seem to "look" right. Worse, you never seem to "feel" right. And then … it feels as if the society you were trying to please suddenly turns on you because now you have an eating disorder, which is a "mental disorder," so now, ironically, you're considered "crazy" by some of the people you were trying to please in the first place!

These illnesses can take years to recover from. If you ever feel suicidal during your recovery, don't face it alone. Even though it may seem more comfortable to keep it to yourself, DON'T! Turn to someone you can trust and open up to them. Seek professional help. You don't have to remain lost in your circumstances — "problems" are temporary. There's an old saying, "Suicide is a permanent solution to a temporary problem." It's true. We know many people who felt suicidal, but gave life another chance only to find the happiness, recovery and fulfillment they were looking for. Realize this: you are precious. You need to give yourself time.

For those who've lost the fight, these deaths are all too real. We know too many people we deeply loved who died from eating disorders, whether through suicide or through medical complications. If you've lost someone special to an eating disorder, join us in honoring their lives and knowing their spirits live on. We know their beautiful spirits continue to surround and guide us as special guardian angels. One of these special guardian angels may even be whispering encouragement in your ear right now, so gently you barely notice. That angel knows your pain, tells you not to give up, and assures you everything will be okay.

Every year, the National Association of Anorexia Nervosa and Associated Disorders (ANAD) hosts a candlelight vigil with the theme *It's better to light a candle than to curse the darkness*. Maria, as clinical director of eating disorders services at Linden Oaks Hospital in Naperville, Illinois, began the tradition of hosting an ANAD candlelight vigil. Attendance at the most recent vigils totaled more than four-hundred-fifty people. Here, those who've lost their lives to eating disorders are remembered. Loved ones speak out to honor the person they've lost and to help others find hope and recovery.

For the last two years, Al, the grieving father of Kim, whom we lovingly remembered in Chapter Seven with her poem *Numb* – has spoken at the vigil. "If only Kim's death could help one person," he says, reminding us how precious life is. The vigil also celebrates the recovery of those who've put eating disorders behind them. We encourage you to host your own candlelight vigil near your home. Contact ANAD for more information at www.ANAD.org.

Forgiveness is the most important part of healing from the death of a loved one who died from an eating disorder. Watching someone you care about struggle with this illness naturally creates anger and helplessness. You may need to forgive your loved one. Hopefully, as time passes, you'll come to understand that the afflicted person didn't intend to get the illness; she/he didn't have control over much of it. You may also need to grant yourself forgiveness, because it's normal to ask, "What could I have done differently?"

Remind yourself that we have little control over a loved one's disorder. Planting a tree, a garden, or other living things can be a cathartic and meaningful remembrance. We know people who used the death of a loved one to bring about good in the world, such as the Aubrey's Song Foundation in Kentucky, an organization that raises money for eating disorder treatment in honor of Aubrey Michelle Clark, who died in 2005 at the age of twenty-two.

RECOVERY TIME

Things to know: the average length of time to recover from an eating disorder is one to five years. Some people may struggle for ten or twenty years before recovering. While battling the disorder, people are often stuck in a major depression and feel isolated and misunderstood. They obsess, lose hope, and become riddled with self-hatred and anxiety – especially when loved ones become frustrated with them. "I can't believe you're still dealing with this!" and "Why don't you just eat!" and "You know what to do, so just do it!" are commonly heard. Those comments only make the sufferer feel others have given up on them.

Loved ones, remember this: your beloved is still here. Sometimes, it's challenging to find them underneath the desperate obsession. Get help for yourself too. Watching someone we love suffer is traumatic. You typically feel helpless, frustrated, and even angry. Fortunately, most ANAD meetings welcome family and friends. Many parents, families, and friends become involved in their own therapy to successfully help a loved one.

If you have an eating disorder, never give up. Know this: you're worth it. You can do it. People have recovered fully after having an eating disorder for a month, a year, five years, ten years, and even more than twenty years. Each recovery is different, because each person's story is unique. As Patrick and Rhonda demonstrated, eating disorders are found in many people, in diverse environments.

So, let's examine the pieces that weave together to make a recovery possible.

What does recovery look like? Recovery looks great. Well, at first maybe not, because the issues the eating disorder masked or helped avoid – especially the F word (Feelings) ... those issues will likely jump out at you full force. Bingeing, purging, restricting eating, over-exercising – each of these behaviors serves to take your attention away from feelings. But relief from painful feelings only fuels the eating disorder. Yes, starve yourself in one area of your life and guess what? You wind up feeding something else in an unhealthy way.

But, through healthy eating, something magical eventually occurs; you unfreeze feelings you possibly didn't even know about.

Amy, a twenty-seven-year-old wife and high school math teacher, writes...

66When I first started to restrict, it wasn't about how much I weighed or how I looked. Instead, restricting gave me a sense of power over the choices I had in life. I was actually proud of the fact that I could restrict. I often thought I was smarter than everyone else because I found a way to live without being dependent upon food. This feeling fueled a drive to continue restricting, which evolved into a horrific restricting cycle that began ruling my life. The hard part was, I was only eight years old.

The eating disorder took on a life of its own by the time I reached high school. Eventually my restricting did become about how I looked. I obsessed about being thin. I went to any and all lengths to reach a certain weight, only to find myself lowering the bar each time. It's hard to admit, but I felt superior to my friends and peers because I knew I had this little secret – a secret that kept me safe. As long as I told no one, I created a world where I held all the power.

Nineteen years passed before I got treatment. My restricting cycle became so severe that it consumed my life. Everything else in the world could have melted away, so long as I was thin. Going to treatment and learning how to re-feed my body proved the hardest thing I've ever done. I had to re-teach my body how to eat. I had to sit with being uncomfortable, praying my doctors were right about how my body would react to food. I had to be patient with my meal plan and trust my dietitian. When I began trusting my treatment team, the cycle finally broke. I was free of an obsession that consumed me since third grade. I'm now proud to say I am in recovery from anorexia and I plan on staying there. **"**

During the early stages of recovery your feelings may be overwhelming, but think about what a blessing it is to once again experience feelings in a healthy way.

Soak this up. You have the right to know, understand, and – most of all – feel your own emotions. This is a vital part of knowing who you are, what you need, and what you want from life.

People who've been in recovery for months or years reveal how much they enjoy, even love, their current lives and say they would never return to the previous existence. Most of them acquired a stellar support system in the form of great friends. They experience happiness and, perhaps most importantly, found deeper meaning in their lives. Recovery is a hard road at first, but the results are priceless.

SEVEN WAYS TO RECOVER FROM AN EATING DISORDER

1. Know Thyself: Get Therapy

Yes, therapy. Every eating disorder is a unique puzzle, including a story about how that puzzle came into being and what kept it glued together. As a person unravels the knots that keep them stuck, therapy can be a huge blessing. But it's important to find the right therapist. Remember, these folks work for you. You need to work with someone who's trustworthy and emotionally safe so you can honestly and openly approach your issues.

What feelings reside underneath an eating disorder? Don't think it's about being a little brat who refuses to eat a sandwich. Many factors play into eating disorders, including challenging life circumstances. And most people aren't aware they're getting an eating disorder. It sneaks up on them.

Twenty-two-year-old Amy loves her boyfriend and her dog now, but here she tells why she had an eating disorder throughout her teens.

> 66As a young girl I lost my mother to lung cancer. I wanted so much to fit in with everyone else, but at nine I was set apart from all the other kids because my mom was gone. Nobody knew how to handle my situation. I always felt so alone. I pretended that losing my mom didn't affect me. I thought I wanted friends, but I really wanted my mom. I believed the only way I could have friends was if I got skinny enough. I struggled through my teen years

with anorexia and experimented with drugs. The treatment I received for my eating disorder and the tender care of my support team helped me through recovery, because they showed me I was valuable. Now that I'm recovered, I can look back and see what helped me beat that skinny bitch Ana(rexia). "

Kristin, a twenty-three-year-old who's in treatment, recovering from seven years of anorexia and bulimia, explains her eating disorder and the problems that can arise with a relapse.

"I'm currently working on building confidence to set appropriate boundaries with my mom and keep myself from falling apart. She's been an alcoholic her entire life. I can't tell you how much harder it is to hear her drunk and slurring her words when I'm healthy, compared to when I'm sick. When I'm sick I can ignore it, because I'm just as in it as she is. But I don't want this for my life. I want so much more. When I speak to her now I feel as though I'm speaking to my mom's alcoholism. I want to shake her and scream, "Where are you? Where have you been?" Her eyes are empty. She looks lost and I feel so alone – as if there's a sinking hole in my chest. I lose my appetite and want to curl up and cry, and entirely shut down. However, I'm learning how to cope, and I'm getting stronger every day. "

And forty-seven-year-old Cheryl, a wife, mother, and excited new grandmother, shares her story.

"When I first lost enough weight to elicit positive and negative attention from others, I began to equate thinness with accomplishment, a specialness

I possessed, and it gave me a sense of power. Being thin, along with the attention I received, became the most important goal of my existence. Prior to becoming thin, I didn't exactly hate my body; I hated myself and my life. I felt I had no self. Being thin gave me a purpose and a false sense of myself. Feeling like you have no self is a terrifying feeling. Finding the answer to the infamous question of "who am I?" and "who am I if not my eating disorder?" became my new focus. I found the answer to these questions is that you and I always have been, and always will be, at the core of our beings. And our cores include love, peace, pureness, beauty, and perfection. No thought, feeling, action, or story can ever change that truth. This is how we were born and what we need to remember as we live. There are many ways to truly connect with and know the "I am," the core, the essence or the true self in us all. **"**

CAUTION: Since eating disorders are invisible to the eye, remember that therapists, support groups, and dieticians aren't able to monitor whether a person is medically safe, stable, or healthy. A physician who's well informed about eating disorders can check the medical condition during recovery. If you have an eating disorder, listen to your body and get help when you don't feel well. Remember the death threat discussed above. It's real. Look out for yourself. Remember that 82 percent of in-patients with eating disorders also had another co-existing full-blown psychiatric diagnosis, the most common being depression, anxiety disorder, obsessive-compulsive disorder, or substance abuse. You may want to talk with a psychiatric specialist about whether medications would help your recovery. Many people have used medication to assist them and make a positive difference in their lives.

2. Support, Support, Support

Try to locate a local support group where you can be heard and understood. Too many people with eating disorders feel isolated and have no one to talk with about the maze they're trapped in. Receiving support allows people to open up to others and be more up front with themselves as well. Some support groups are open to family and friends, while others are reserved for people with eating disorders. ANAD, NEDA (the National Eating Disorders Association), EDA (Eating Disorders Anonymous) and OA (Overeaters Anonymous) offer free support groups. Investigate until you find the right place for you.

Two Things to Watch Out For in Support Groups:

- Eating disorders are contagious. Make sure participants aren't focusing on complaining and feeling victimized. At this time in your life, it's vital to surround yourself with positive people. If you discover people being too negative or so ingrained with their disorders that it somehow triggers you, confront the group and ask if people are willing to work together to make the group experience more recovery-focused. If this isn't well received, then feel free to look around for another group, or contact one of the organizations listed in this chapter and start your own. Groups work best when everyone is committed to recovery and holding themselves accountable.

- Some 12-step recovery models are challenging when applied to eating disorders. Alcoholics can abstain from alcohol, but how can a person who's addicted to eating abstain from food? Actually, abstaining from eating *is* the unhealthy goal of anorexia. To deal with this dilemma, some treatment models designate white sugar and white flour as the addiction to abstain from. Unfortunately, we've found this well-meaning technique feeds right into the rigid eating disorder mindset. Don't avoid large food groups as part of your recovery. Everything in moderation, remember? What you need to abstain from is restricting food, bingeing, purging, compulsive over-exercising, body-checking, socially isolating, lying, and all other eating disorder behaviors. *Remember: Restricting is always the core behavior.* No one wants to engage in the other behaviors, but they don't want to give up restricting either. You have to give up restricting to recover and ultimately gain control of your eating.

3. The Food Police: Eating Disorder Dieticians, a Special Breed

Perhaps you're saying, "I don't need a dietician, I already know everything about nutrition." We're sure you do. You could write a textbook about good eating – as long as it discusses what *someone else* is supposed to eat. Last time we checked, you were a bit fearful and hesitant about applying it to yourself, which is why we call this an eating disorder. When you have an eating disorder, you don't always use good judgment about your own nutrition. Or a parent may say, "We don't need to pay a dietician to tell her what she already knows she needs to do." Even if you've been told what to eat and you know certain eating disorder behaviors aren't healthy for you, you may still require step-by-step assistance and structure so you feel safe during recovery.

We'd love for you to eat when you're hungry and stop when you're full. We'd also love for you to eat food you love – in moderation. But if you have an eating disorder, you may be a few steps away from these ideals. Find a program or a dietician who understands how to structure a meal plan for your specific needs. Using the Food Pyramid exchange system, you could remind your body about normal eating again. The challenge for people with eating disorders is that they usually lose sight of their hunger and fullness cues. If this is the case, you could benefit from a dietician to guide you with "mechanical eating" as you give your body the time it needs to learn to listen to itself once again.

People in recovery have reported it takes as long as six months to a year to restore the body's natural hunger and fullness cues, so keep following your plan until you can do it on your own. Your dietician will help you transition from your meal plan to intuitive eating when you both agree the time is right. The other benefit of working with a dietician is that you can work on your list of good foods and bad foods, so that over time you'll eat all foods you desire in moderation. Finally, your dietician will monitor your weight for you and help you feel safe as you change food habits. This allows you to make sure your meal plan is the correct one for you, without having to deal with seeing your weight. Of course you'll need to look around for a dietician with special training in eating disorders. Getting a dietician who wants you to count calories or focuses on how you need to restrict fats and carbs will just feed into the problem.

4. Express Yourself

Oh, let us count the ways. For starters, consider writing. If you have an eating disorder travel back in time. Write your autobiography and create a timeline about your life. Connect different ages to moods, significant negative and positive events, and symptoms of an eating disorder, depression, and anxiety. This will help you unravel the eating disorder and find the real *you* again. You may be surprised at how an old scenario of being teased, having someone mention your weight, or an event you have never talked about before may be a factor in how this eating disorder took over your life. Take note of other forms of expression that can be cathartic.

Conversation. Try talking things over openly in therapy or with friends and family; let things out instead of keeping them in all the time.

Movement. Get in touch with your body through exercise. Try yoga, dance, stretching, walking, swimming, Pilates – the list goes on, right? Movement reminds you that your body is an instrument. And remember, the idea is to move your body in a respectful, positive way. Don't do it for the sole purpose of burning calories. Shake it up. Shake up the joy hidden inside.

Music is healing. Sing at the top of your lungs (in the shower or in your car.) Perhaps you like to write music or play an instrument. Listening to music is often cathartic, especially when you relate to the songs. One caution: avoid listening to only negative and depressing songs. Sure, if you were depressed it would feel false to avoid sad music. But if that's all you listen to, you'll soon find yourself spinning into a vortex of greater depression. Be sure you insert joyful, hopeful, fun songs into your playlist.

Art. Thirty-two-year-old Heather, a wife, mother of four, and art therapist, explains, "I expressed every feeling and emotion through art making. The eating disorder still wanted control and I had many slips, but all the while I worked on my art. It became something I could be known for other than being the girl with the eating disorder."

5. Exposure Therapy

These treatments expose people to things they would normally fear and avoid. For those suffering from eating disorders, this consists of eating certain feared foods and becoming aware of the body. Examples include eating in restaurants, going grocery shopping, looking in the mirror, wearing a bathing suit at a pool, touching one's body, and looking at a personal photograph. Other exposure therapies don't target eating disorders directly, but attack issues surrounding and supporting the disorder. These include, reaching out for help instead of isolating; sitting with, smelling, and touching foods you may be frightened to eat; dealing with emotion and trauma issues; spending less time on homework, cleaning, or exercise (for you perfectionists); and eating what the family eats (instead of some special type of safe food).

If your natural reaction to that is, "No way, those are too scary!" then you just demonstrated you need exposure therapy. Taking steps toward incorporating positive eating and body image into your life is the best way to replace a life ridden with fear. Doing these frightening activities with trusted friends, family, and treatment team members helps take away the fear. Give yourself credit for every step you take.

6. Get Soul

When you have an eating disorder, the SBM attempts to take over, and you feel as though you've been taken hostage. Your soul feels crushed and you may temporarily lose sight of your heart's desires and true values.

Thirty-one-year-old Meghan was only recently able to wear one of the most important symbols of her treasured family.

> **❝**I put my wedding rings on for the first time in over two years this past week. What was once a symbol of eternal love with my husband had become a symbol of my eating disorder. If those rings fit on my finger, I was still fat. How could something so precious to me turn into something so scary? Nothing is too sacred for an eating disorder to attack. But I fought back and won. Now I wear my rings not with fear, but with trust, honesty, and respect for my new life in recovery.**❞**

Spiritual healing is crucial to recovery, because it answers the question "Why recover?" Twenty-two-year old Erica, a theology major, helps us link all the spiritual pieces together.

> **❝**Throughout the course of my struggle with anorexia, I couldn't help but feel God had somehow let me slip through His fingers. He wasn't paying attention, and I had fallen hard. Like glass, I shattered into a million pieces. It wasn't until my recovery that I realized God was indeed paying attention, and He was there every step of the way.

He wept with me when I fell. He swept up all the
tiny pieces and one-by-one He helped me glue
them back together. God used those jagged pieces
of me to create a mosaic much more beautiful
than anything I could have ever been if I hadn't
experienced the fall and the shattering. And
while it's true that some pieces don't fit together
perfectly, I like to think of the tiny cracks as
beautiful opportunities for the light that's now in
me to shine through for others to see. **99**

7. "Service, Please!"

True story. One night, long ago, author Greg was asleep. In a
dream, he was busy working at a barista in a popular coffeehouse/
bookstore in his town. After making a few coffee drinks, he turned
around to tend to the next customer. Imagine his surprise when he
found Jesus standing there. (Yes. *The* Jesus – white robe, sandals, nice
eyes, and everything.) Curiously, Greg remained calm. Then, Jesus
tapped the counter gently with his forefinger and said, "I'd like some
service, please."

Which brings us to the next chapter...

By the Numbers

12 million: the number of people in the United States diagnosed with anorexia or bulimia nervosa.

25 million: the number of people who suffer from binge-eating disorder.

45/25: the percentage of dieting women and men on any given day.

50: the percentage of third, fourth, and fifth grade boys and girls who are dissatisfied with their bodies. The vast majority think they're too fat.

21: the percentage of five-year-olds who are dissatisfied with their bodies and think they're fat.

81: the percentage of ten-year-olds afraid of being fat.

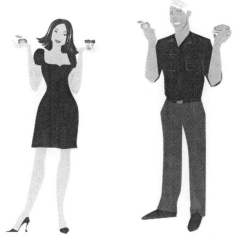

"A few weeks ago I picked up a child from the street, and from the face I could see that little child was hungry. I didn't know how many days that little one had not eaten. So I gave her a piece of bread, and the little one took the bread and, crumb by crumb, started eating it. I said to her, 'Eat, eat the bread. You are hungry.' And the little one looked at me and said, 'I am afraid. When the bread will be finished, I will be hungry again.'"

—Mother Teresa, from *No Greater Love*

Chapter Ten
Shut Up, And Go Do Some Service

THERE'S A GREAT CONTRAST BETWEEN what's really important in life, and what society values. Think about our cultural emphasis on thinness. Certain books ask us to imagine how cool we'd be if we were thin enough to look awesome in a thong when we walk down the street. Really? Think about that. Why do we accept that crap? What does it say about a society that continually perpetuates the illusion that externals are more important than the interior package, when intrinsically we know the opposite is true.

Yes, we buy into these poisonous ideas. We read and absorb them. We take in mental empty calories passed down to us by mass media, portions of the medical system, and snarky skinny bitches, all of whom pressure people into thinking they must be ultrathin to be acceptable.

Again, Laura, the thirty-one-year-old documentary filmmaker who's been recovered from her eating disorder for six years, proudly tells us...

66 Thinness does not solve anything. It doesn't solve wars, violence against women, or guns in schools, and it definitely doesn't solve world hunger. I knew, more or less, when I had anorexia that thinness would not solve any of these things, but I mistakenly thought it would solve my personal and emotional problems – my own issues. But it didn't. Eventually, the thing that solved my own personal and emotional problems was learning to communicate my feelings to myself and others. Honestly, that was the only thing I've ever tried that actually worked. And it didn't take thinness to learn how to be emotional and communicate my emotions. Now, if only the people running countries today could learn how to communicate better to solve their problems. 99

When we're obsessed with food and weight, we're much like a hamster on a little wheel, running around, burning energy, and ultimately going nowhere. We use our precious time, energy, and life force to go in (emotional) circles, chasing nothing of importance. We know you're hungry for something better. And if you've absorbed anything from reading this book, you'll know that you no longer need to be bullied into thinking your body has to be a certain size to fit in. Ask yourself what group you're trying to fit into, because the only skinny thing found in the groups we all think we want to be a part of is meaningful conversation.

We say, "Shut up! We have better things to do!" Like eat. We need to nourish ourselves so we can have the energy – remember, eating food gives you energy – to make this world a better place in some way. Take that in. If you're too busy obsessing about how much chocolate syrup you had on your ice cream or why your jeans are always tight, then how much time can you devote to giving back to your community and beyond?

The moment you give something back to the world is the moment you begin to heal.

Several years ago, Maria was reflecting on the actual value of food. After helping create a successful eating disorder program at Linden Oaks Hospital in Naperville, Illinois, and seeing dozens of young girls, women, boys, and men go through treatment, she wondered what else could be done to help people understand the real value of food.

"What is food and eating really about?" she asked herself. The answer: food is a life or death matter. But why does modern society fail to take it seriously? Then she had an insight. "If you want to know what the value of food is, you need to spend time with the hungry."

Well, that was a gorgeous cherry to place atop the cake.

Maria began designing and implementing this idea into a program to augment her other eating disorder treatments. She realized people with eating disorders are basically hungry. They carry a myriad of issues and emotions wrapped up in their relationship with food. People who self-starve have trained themselves to not even recognize hunger. Yet, many people in the world are starving because they don't have access to food. What would happen if these two groups met?

That's when the magic happened.

Maria dubbed her program Real Meals and incorporated the idea into a treatment plan that let her eating disorders patients participate in a field trip outing to feed the homeless at a local community shelter. The project began with a group discussion about world hunger. Patients shared their thoughts about starvation and the poverty that existed around them. The next step was to create a menu and grocery list, and then venture to the grocery store to shop for the foods needed to create meals for the homeless.

Even before the meals were made, something unexpected and incredibly cathartic took place.

Shopping for the groceries morphed into another kind of intervention. Maria soon reconfirmed what she'd already learned: eating disorder patients were often overwhelmed inside a grocery store and frightened to buy certain foods. We're talking things like ground beef, butter, and pasta to serve the group of homeless people who'd arrive for the meal. If the patients were told, "Hey, let's go buy a huge amount of ground beef, butter, and pasta to feed you guys tonight, okay?" there wouldn't be any takers. But knowing they were going to feed the hungry brought motivation to these people who feared food. They dashed around the store *joyfully* gathering ingredients.

The next stop – the kitchen at the homeless shelter. There, everyone worked with huge quantities of food as they prepared the meal. Her heart filled with hope, Maria took a step back and watched the dozen or so patients in her program work together. Those who had major issues about even touching food got right in there – getting their hands dirty with something (food) they'd been struggling to learn to embrace.

And then, the patients came face to face with the hungry. One by one, homeless men and women poured into the basement of the local church. And one by one, the eating disorders patients saw they had something in common with them: hunger. The difference? The homeless didn't purposely restrict their food intake.

Have you ever seen true hunger? It's the pained, yet grateful look in someone's eyes as they wait in a long line to take whatever food is offered. There's no concern about fat content, carbohydrates, or whether there's butter in the sauce. No one frets about counting calories. No. There, in those food lines, was a completely different approach to the meaning and value of food – we all need it to survive.

In this intervention, the patients not only prepared the food, they served it, and then sat among the guests and ate with them. Remember, if these same patients were asked to eat this same food at dinner "just because," there would be no takers. But since they were doing it to serve others, suddenly they could partake and feel happy. At one meal, a patient was so frightened about eating what was on her plate that tears trickled down her face. The homeless man sitting next to her noticed. He stopped eating his meal for a moment and tried to comfort her. "I hate to see someone sad," the homeless man said. More tears. As the man reassured her, she was able to finish her meal.

Time for dessert. (Oh, dear!) Yes. They had dessert, served with enthusiasm. And the eating disorders patients consumed their servings, too.

After clean-up, the patients prepared bag lunches for the homeless, so they'd have a meal the following day – and then it was time to process what had just unfolded.

The group sat together to discuss their feelings and experiences during the evening. The hope was to illuminate the true meaning of food and hunger and help those with eating disorders see a new perspective on the things keeping them stuck. The homeless people didn't count calories. They didn't worry if the food would give them love handles. They were grateful to have any food.

Twenty-four-year-old Erin and nineteen-year-old Ari are both fully recovered from their eating disorders. Both of them have participated in Real Meals. Erin shares her story.

66 Led by our therapists and dieticians, we shopped for, prepared, and served a meal to the homeless. We then sat and ate with them. We talked to the homeless about where they were from and heard their stories. Everyone in that room had a story. I remember being struck by the number of people coming in for the meal. A lot of them didn't look homeless – they were every age and race, both sexes, and even children. Along the same lines, a lot of us didn't look like we had eating disorders – we're every age, every race, and both sexes, including children. My eyes were opened to a new level of awareness. At that point in treatment, I would normally feel a lot of anxiety about the pizza and ice cream sundae meal we were having. But that night, I had no anxiety. Nothing about my

eating disorder mattered because I was involved in something more important and real. I was eating with people who didn't have a choice about being hungry. They were grateful to us for the food and conversation, and I was grateful to them for lessons learned. We were brought together by hunger, but I can tell you no one left hungry that night. For the first time in a long time I didn't feel guilty for not being hungry. I felt satisfied.**99**

Ari says that when she was thirteen years old, she was doing different activities than most of her other friends in junior high school.

66I was being hospitalized for anorexia nervosa for the third time. I'd been battling and suffering from my disease for three years at that point. My eating disorder locked me into being centered around myself. I constantly wanted to take care of everyone else, but I spared no one's feelings if they got in the way of doing a behavior. Because my people-pleasing mentality was firmly contradicted by my selfish and self-destructive behavior, I found myself disconnected from who I was. While I was hospitalized at Linden Oaks, we did a feeding-the-homeless excursion. Our group went to the grocery store to buy food we would use to make a meal, and later eat with people who desperately needed it. In retrospect, this was the perfect way to confuse us into figuring out who we really were and what we wanted. One thing I had in common with every person in our group was a strong desire to help those in need. Seeing patients who were often brought to tears by the thought of eating a meal become excited to buy ingredients for the very meal they usually feared, was inspirational. Although several girls had conflicting emotions, it brought out the strength in all of us. At least for that one night the food had greater meaning and purpose.

After preparing and serving the meal, we finally sat down to eat with our new friends. That meal was a feat for everyone sitting at the table, but for different reasons. Seeing the gratitude of people who received something I'd taken for granted gave me a new perspective that helped me during my weakest times. Altruism has been an enormous facet of my recovery. When I was sick I truly couldn't help others because my disease kept me selfish and too sick to give myself to others. Now, six years later I am fully recovered from my eating disorder. It's hard to say how much one single activity or therapy session makes or breaks a recovery process, but I can confidently say that without connecting with the giving part of myself, I could not be where I am today. My life and my recovery were shaped by goals I wouldn't have made for myself if I hadn't seen with my own eyes the impact I could make. "

THREE THINGS YOU CAN DO TO GET OUT OF YOUR HEAD, OUT OF PAIN, AND RECOVER FROM FOOD AND WEIGHT ISSUES

1. Volunteer

Head to a local food pantry or homeless shelter and spend time getting to know what hunger truly is. This will help you understand the true value of food. But don't stop there. Think of other things – other needy people in your community and around the world. Find out how you can serve them. Feel free to create your own opportunities to serve. The bottom line: you'll truly see that when you help others, it all comes back to you. It's one thing to sit around in a support group trying convince yourself you're a good person. It's another thing to go out and *show* how great you are. When you see your own hands helping others, you can't easily dismiss the evidence. This is not a theoretical discussion. It's real. It's a fact that can't be disputed. Serving others heals those you serve, and you. As you enter into this phase of serving, keep a journal and record your thoughts. Watch yourself become less concerned with every detail about your body and eating. Soon, you'll replace society-driven concerns with things that are truly meaningful. You'll discover things about yourself that make you excited to live and be around others.

2. Bring Sexy Back

Are you tired of people telling you the only sexy thing is a perfect body? Each person is sexy in his or her own way, and we have a right to feel that way. We need to push back on cultural bullying. As in saying "Shut up!"

Things we find sexy:
- listening when people talk,
- caring about others,
- working for peace in your family and life,
- sporting intelligent views on world issues,
- great dance moves,
- a fine voice,
- forgiveness (nothing better, really),
- that sparkle in your eye,
- a hilarious, yet warm, sense of humor, and
- knowing how to prepare a tax return.

What do you want from a relationship – a hot body, or amazing conversation with someone you trust and love? If you said a hot bod, we say, "Shut up!" So, let's start fighting back against our thin-obsessed culture and cultivate deeper meaning in our lives.

3. Fight Back/Speak Up

One day in Maria's eating disorders program, one of her patients said, "I agree with everything you're saying. You're right. But soon I'll have to leave the hospital and go back into a world that tells me I'm wrong and something's wrong with me. I'm scared!"

But fear needn't hold us back from speaking out for justice. By banding together and insisting thin is *not* in, we send a ripple effect into the world. We educate. We remind ourselves and others that all sizes and shapes are indeed beautiful, sexy, and healthy.

Nicole, a nineteen-year-old college student, boldly recovered from her eating disorder. We found her words inspiring.

> **"**For the past seven years I would stare down the candles on the birthday cake. I wouldn't eat and make the same wish before blowing them out, "Please let me reach my goal weight before my next birthday." Everyone would smile and cheer once the candles were blown out, but the hissing voice of my eating disorder drowned out their wishes. The truth is, I never reached a goal weight because there was no such thing. When you finally get there, you find yourself wanting lower. That goal weight was the only solid thing in my life, which was ironic because of how often that number changed. Knowing that maybe I would be "x" pounds lighter by my next birthday was the only thing keeping me alive. That was true, but at the same time it was killing me. Things have begun to change now. For the first time in the past seven years, I am fighting. This year I will have my cake and eat it, too!**"**

And there you have it. Your "Shut Up, Skinny Bitches!" manifesto; a delicious reminder to eat well, play, feel your emotions, embrace the size you are, and best of all, spread love through doing service. Each of us has an impact on the world, whether we realize it or not. If you walk away with anything after reading this book, we hope it's a combination of one of the following:

1. You're fine just the way you are – nothing is wrong with you or your size.

2. You have the power within you to recognize your hunger and fullness cues. Food is not something you should fear, but something to manage (like a checking account) and yes, you can manage it. And...

3. It's okay to eat a cheeseburger or piece of chocolate cake – more often than you think.

In the meantime, we wish you love and acceptance of your body, your whole self, and others around you.

Now ... go eat something!

SERVICE, PLEASE!

"Altruism has been an enormous facet of my recovery. When I was sick I truly couldn't help others because my disease kept me focused on my own concerns and too sick to give myself to others."

—Ari

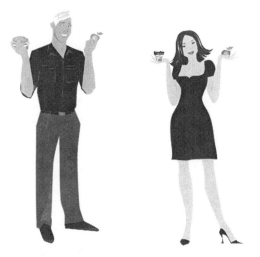

"They may be bitches, but they are skinny bitches."

—*Skinny Bitch/* back cover

Epilogue
Our Savory Critique of the Book 'Skinny Bitch'

YEAH, WE SAID WE WEREN'T SINGLING OUT the book *Skinny Bitch*, and we're not. But we couldn't pass up delivering a book review of our own. After all, we love food *and* have strong opinions. But first, a story.

One day Maria was looking forward to a counseling session with Haley. At 17, Haley's role in the family had been taking care of everyone but herself, and it finally caught up with her. She developed anorexia nervosa. Her first two counseling sessions went well. She was working on giving up her lists of good foods and bad foods, challenging herself to overcome her fear of eating, and even considering weight gain. She felt safe and her attitude was positive.

But the moment Haley walked through the door that day, Maria knew something had happened. Haley appeared tense, angry, and confused, as though she no longer felt safe. Then Maria noticed

Haley's bony hand clutching a little book. Maria asked her what she was holding, and the words "Skinny Bitch" came into view. That introduction to the book made Maria realize the message to be thin is like a cancer running rampant in our society.

After the Haley incident we read *Skinny Bitch* by Rory Freedman and Kim Barnouin. Here's our critique of the book. We deliver it to help anyone who feels stuck about their size, weight, appearance, eating habits, or self-esteem. We want you to come to better terms with loving yourselves and loving food, too.

Now, let's debunk a gaggle of myths we found in the book.

You must be thin to be happy.

Shut Up! The book *Skinny Bitch* begins like this, "Are you sick and tired of being fat? Good. If you can't take one more day of self-loathing, you're ready to get skinny."

We've repeatedly seen how believing happiness, love, and all good things in life will arrive *only* when you lose weight is a recipe for unhappiness. We're thinking you guys are smart cookies – that you don't stand for discrimination against people because of skin color or religion. So, think about it. Why is it okay to believe thin people are superior to those who are less thin? This type of thinking is justified in the book, because the perception is that heavier people are responsible for their condition. If only they didn't eat so much of the wrong foods, they wouldn't be so fat. Weight loss doesn't solve self-esteem issues. Love yourself for who you are!

You must allow yourself to be spoken to harshly, especially if you're overweight, which we all are because apparently, everyone needs to lose weight, right?

Nope. In the guise of being a friendly girlfriend, *Skinny Bitch* cuts everyone down to size. The book calls the reader a "gluttonous pig," a "moron," a "shithead," a "cheap asshole" and, excuse our language, dear reader, a "pussy." (Sorry!) We'd say the authors swear like sailors, but the sailors we know only speak respectfully to others. In fact, we don't know anybody who uses language that foul. But the book tries to come across as cute, as though the authors are skinny girlfriends just trying to reach out to readers, because, well, those poor readers haven't figured out how to be gorgeous? (Gee, no thank you.)

We noticed millions of people purchased the book. They were called all the names listed here, yet they kept reading. We wondered why folks allowed themselves to be spoken to so rudely. Later, we realized readers might justify this kind of treatment by saying, "Well, I don't normally like to be called a pussy, but these guys are my friends, and since I'm fat they're just trying to motivate me so I can slim down and finally be acceptable in the world."

Listen up. Don't let anyone talk to you that way – including yourself. It's not good for your self-esteem.

Are we fat pigs?

Not Even! Who are all these fat, gluttonous pigs so often cited in *Skinny Bitch*? Apparently every reader is one, but some of the readers must be normal weight, or even underweight. Haley was underweight when she read the book, but it made her feel like a moron with gross vices. She became anxious, fearful, and her self-esteem plummeted as she tried to be as special as a skinny bitch. No mention is made of what you're supposed to weigh to fit in with the people who exist in the *Skinny Bitch* universe. In our opinion, the book's real message is this: You Can Never Be Thin Enough!

It's not a diet book!

If it looks like a diet book and reads like one, then guess what? It's a diet book.

Skinny Bitch claims it is not a diet book, but it tells you what to expect in the first month of acquiring the lifestyle. "Chances are, there will be times you feel deprived, angry, overwhelmed, and frustrated. But these few, fleeting moments will all be worthwhile once you are skinny."

Yeah, that actually sounds like how any of us feel the moment we start this thing called – A DIET!

Most people today understand that diets fail. So, now they're using a new word for dieting: lifestyle. Lifestyle could be a term used for little changes that are powerful and relatively easy to implement, which could do a world of good and not impair your quality of life. This might include adopting a fun exercise plan into your life, or eating a bit less sugar and more fresh vegetables. But when you're given strict rules on what and how to eat, we call that a diet. And when you're told to realize you're a "fat, bloated, gluttonous pig" when you don't follow those rules, well, we just call that dieting hell.

Milk does not do a body good.

Really? Skinny Bitch readers are warned to avoid eating dairy products, which the author says cause cancer, obesity, and osteoporosis. Readers are assured of the following if they give up milk and dairy products. "You will pee in your pants when you see how much weight you lose from giving up dairy.

Milk = fat,

Butter = fat,

Cheese = fat.

People who think these products can be low fat or fat free are fucking morons."

Maybe you should hold off on peeing in your pants for a second. When we checked the source of the book's information, it was "highly scientific" – milksucks.com.

Perhaps you'd be more comfortable with articles found in research journals. A 2004 study in *Osteoporosis International* cites that milk improved the bone mineral density in children to help them accomplish lifelong protection against hip and vertebral fractures. Then there's the *International Journal of Epidemiology*, which in 2005 recommended milk to protect against vascular disease (particularly its powerful reduction of blood pressure), protection against diabetes and colon cancer, and milk's role in helping "ensure the full potential growth of children." The latter study also found the jury is out on milk's role in body weight, as studies have shown that milk helps with weight loss and weight gain.

Here's an idea. How about if we just have milk in moderation?

You simply must give up meat, especially red meat.

Hold off on that... With a chapter title like "The dead, rotting decomposing flesh diet," it's easy to tell the authors don't want people to eat meat. "You will be a fat, unhealthy, bloated pig if you live this way," the book warns. The authors seem to have various reasons why we're total morons if we eat meat. This also caught our attention: "Many meat eaters credit eating meat for our evolution from cavemen into what we are now. Even if this were the case and eating meat did help us evolve, look at what we evolved from. We looked like friggin' apes and had massive heads, strong jaws, and brute strength. Maybe back then we were supposed to eat meat. But the last time we checked, we weren't cavemen anymore."

Cross our hearts – we didn't change a word. The book actually said that.

These authors observe we don't have all of the characteristics of carnivores, so therefore we're not meant to eat meat. Actually, humans seem to share many characteristics of omnivores, who eat a little bit of everything, in moderation, of course. Michael Murray's *Encyclopedia of Healing Foods* offers thorough research evaluations that conclude consuming fish and meat is optimal for our diets to get enough protein and all of the essential amino acids the human body requires.

And the *International Journal of Cancer* in 2003 reported that after studying forty-eight thousand American women over eighteen years of age, meat consumption did not increase risk of breast cancer.

Give up your gross vices, now.

On Second Thought... According to *Skinny Bitch*, if you want to be thin, "the first thing you need to do is give up your gross vices." And what are these so-evil habits? Alcohol, coffee, junk food, smoking, and all over-the-counter medications. Sugar is "the devil," while coffee is "for pussies." And alcohol, the book claims, causes the following medical problem: bloated fat pig syndrome. (Was that from a medical school textbook?)

Actually, The National Cancer Institute states no risk for women who have one drink of alcohol a day, and men who have two. Maybe it's time to have a cosmo and lighten up a little? While everyone agrees smoking is harmful to your health and there are many reasons to quit, you definitely won't lose weight by stopping. You won't lose a pound if you refuse to take over-the-counter medications, either. And how does coffee cause weight gain? A cup of coffee contains two calories. The American Chemical Society proclaims coffee is the number one source of antioxidants in the United States. It's actually good for you. So sip your fat-free, soy, chai lattes if you must. We'd rather be dead than not have our morning coffee.

As for sugar and junk food, again we say – everything in moderation. Even the book notes how obsessed you'll be with the food you try to cut out of your diet. Oh, but don't worry – readers are told they're allowed to eat "delicious" whole-wheat junk food instead. No thanks. Back off. Having a normal serving of the food we crave and enjoy will prevent a futile cycle of restricting and binging.

Working out decreases appetite.

What? "...working out tends to keep our junk food cravings and elephant appetites at bay," *Skinny Bitch* assures readers. In what universe? Here on Earth, it's well known that when you work out your nutritional needs increase and you become hungrier.

Addiction specialists at work.

Hardly. But judging from what we read, we think the authors are trying to sound like addiction specialists. *Skinny Bitch* informs readers that they are food addicts, and powerless over their addiction. Not to worry, the book lists the cure for addiction – yes, the one man has been searching for all these years. For overcoming addiction, the book says, "Bitch-slap it, and get a hold of yourself."

Reading between the lines, a food addict seems to be someone who actually enjoys eating foods that don't consist of whole-wheat, bulgur, or tofu. The advice we read told us to not "...indulge in a vice item, you might go off the deep end. It is well known in Alcoholics Anonymous that you're only one drink away from your next drunk." The book states, "We just want to impress upon you that it is very easy to obliterate all your progress with one bite, sip, or puff."

Basically, the book insists on avoiding "non-healthy" foods for the rest of one's life.

Here's what *we* want you to do. Eat foods you love. Avoid blacklisting any foods. Enjoy all foods in moderation, and love yourself and your body, for the rest of your life.

Oh, it's just fun and games, Part I

Shut up, and eat! The book *Skinny Bitch* sports a P.S. on the final pages that read, "We couldn't really care less about being skinny." This, after repeatedly suggesting readers do everything they can to be skinny? This is like purposely going to the bathroom on someone's front lawn, and then saying "Ooops. I really didn't mean to do that."

That P.S. doesn't erase one of the book's primary messages: it's superior to be skinny. Compared to all the other messages in the read, the P.S. feels hollow.

Oh, it's just fun and games, Part II

Keep Eating! In our opinion, the most frightening aspect of the book *Skinny Bitch* is the way it feeds into several problems commonly seen in anorexia and bulimia nervosa. The book says, "... shut the fuck up, look at an inspirational picture of a skinny bitch, and clean out your refrigerator." People with eating disorders commonly use this type of thinspiration as a motivation to avoid eating.

The book tells readers what foods are acceptable to eat. It teaches readers a number of ways to distract themselves from hunger, such as brushing one's teeth. The book suggests waiting to eat breakfast until there is real hunger, so, "you'll grow to love that empty feeling in your stomach."

"When you do eat, the breakfast of skinny bitches is organic fruit," the book later notes on page 142. "This may seem light in comparison to your previous bagel or eggs or cereal. But again, once you adapt, you will be totally fulfilled by fruit. Eat one piece (serving) slowly. After a period of time – perhaps ten minutes or so – when you feel hungry, eat another piece, slowly. When you feel hungry again, eat one more. Breakfast is over."

This type of thinking could come right out of the mind of someone suffering from anorexia.

Another way the book helps spawn eating disorders is by encouraging readers to fast. Readers receive brownie points by "willingly abstaining from food," the authors note on page 131. They claim, "For more than five thousand years, fasting has been used as a healthy method of weight loss." And, "Fasts can last anywhere from twenty-four hours to ten days or more."

Do we even need to comment here?

Fasting, even by skipping one meal, has NEVER been a healthy method of weight loss. In fact, the 2007 *EAT-II* long-term study of teens found those who fasted actually *gained* weight over time. When you don't feed yourself, you cause your body to basically eat itself, consuming your organs and muscle, including the heart muscle. Obviously, this encourages anorexia nervosa. Fasting is an unhealthy practice that doesn't even promote weight loss.

The other reason fasting was encouraged is to supposedly cleanse your system. Your body already has a way to cleanse itself – we call it going to the bathroom. That's the body's excellent way of eliminating toxic chemicals and waste. The body already knows how to do this naturally, every day.

As if that isn't enough, we found one more thing in the book that promotes unhealthy eating and generates the thought patterns found in serious conditions like anorexia and bulimia nervosa: donating blood. "Donate blood. You can save a life and lose weight at the same time."

Our jaws dropped when we read that. Fortunately, because our mouths were open, we happily reached for some delectable food to nibble on.

Care to join us?

End Notes

Chapter Two
"The Soft Science of Dietary Fat," Science, 30 March, vol. 291 no. 5513, 2536-2545. Taubes, Gary (2001).

"The relationship between dieting and weight change among preadolescents and adolescents." Pediatrics, 112: 900-6. Field, A.E., Austin, S.B., Taylor, C.B, et. al (2003).

"Dieting: Does it really work?" American Psychologist, 62, April, 2007, 220-233. Mann, T. (2007)

"Why does dieting predict weight gain in adolescents?" Findings from Project EAT II: A 5-year longitudinal study. Journal of the American Dietetic Association, March; 107 (3): 448-55. Neumark-Sztainer, D., Wall, M., Haines, J., Story, M. & Eisenberg, M.E. (2007).

"Prevention of obesity and eating disorders: a consideration of shared risk factors." Health Education Research, 21 (6): 770-782. Haines, J & Neumark-Sztainer, D. (2006).

"News from the Women's Health Initiative: Reducing Total Fat Intake May Have Small Effect on Risk of Breast Cancer, No Effect on Risk of Colorectal Cancer, Heart Disease or Stroke." National Institutes of Health, http://www.nih.gov.

National Institute of Health, (2006).

"The Myth of the Low-fat diet." Burne, J. Health: (2010). (mindbodyhealth.com/lowfatdietmyth.htm)

"Psychosocial Factors and Cardiovascular Diseases." Annual Review of Public Health, 26: 469-500. Everson-Rose, S.A. & Lewis, T.T. (2005).

"Overweight, obesity and mortality in a large prospective cohort of persons 50-71 years old." New England Journal of Medicine, 355: 763 Adams, K.F, Schatzkin, A., Harris, T.B., Kipinis,V., Mouw, T., Ballard-Barbash, R., Hollenbeck, A. & Leitzmann, M.F. (2006).

"Guidelines for Healthy Weight." New England Journal of Medicine, 341: 427-434. Willett, W.C., Dietz, W.H & Colditz, G.A. (1999).

The relationship between low cardiorespiratory fitness and mortality in normal weight, overweight and obese men. Journal of the American Medical Association, 282: 1547-1553. G. Hu, Wei, M, Kampert, J.B., Barlow, C.E., et. al (1999).

American Journal of Cardiology, 15 January 2010, Vol. 105, Issue 2, Pages 192-197.

The Encyclopedia of Healing Foods. NY, Atria Books. Murray, M. (2005).

Aerobic Center Longitudinal Study (1999).

"'Happy' or 'Positive' people observed to have fewer heart attacks, data show. Columbia University Medical Center (2010).

"Not always harmful to health to be overweight." The Medical News, 26, June, 2006, 14:53. Doctoral Dissertations of Linn Kennedy and Susanna Calling from Lin University in Sweden.

"Chocolate consumption in relation to blood pressure and risk of cardiovascular disease in German adults." European Heart Journal, 30(24):2951. Brian Buijsse, Cornelia Weikert, Dagmar Drogan, Manuela Bergmann and Heiner Boeing (2010).

Chapter Three
"The nutritional source: Carbohydrates: Good carbs guide the way." 2010 Harvard School of Public Health.

"Time to value milk." International Journal of Epidemiology, 34 (5). 1160-1162. Elwood, P.C. (2005).

"Self-reported vegetarianism may be a marker for college women at risk for disordered eating." Sheree A. Klopp, MS, RD, Cynthia J. Heiss. PhD, Heather S. Smith, MS. Journal of the American Dietetic Association. 2003 Vol. 103, Issue 6.

Chapter Four
"Cardio respiratory Fitness as a Quantitative Predictor of All-Cause Mortality and Cardiovascular Events in Healthy Men and Women—A Meta-analysis." Satoru Kodama, MD, PhD; Kazumi Saito, MD, PhD; Shiro Tanaka, PhD; Miho Maki, MS; Yoko Yachi, RD, MS; Mihoko Asumi, MS; Ayumi Sugawara, RD; Kumiko Totsuka, RD; Hitoshi Shimano, MD, PhD; Yasuo Ohashi, PhD; Nobuhiro Yamada, MD, PhD; Hirohito Sone, MD, PhD JAMA. 2009;301(19):2024-2035.)

"Joint effects of physical activity, body mass index, waist circumference and waist-to-hip ratio with the risk of cardiovascular disease among middle-aged Finnish men and women." Gang Hua, Jaakko Tuomilehtoa, Karri Silventoinenb, Nöel Barengoc and Pekka Jousilahtia, European Heart Journal (2004) 25 (24): 2212-2219.

"Relationship of Physical Fitness vs Body Mass Index With Coronary Artery Disease and Cardiovascular Events in Women." Timothy R. Wessel, MD; Christopher B. Arant, MD; Marian B. Olson, MS; B. Delia Johnson, PhD; Steven E. Reis, MD; Barry L. Sharaf, MD; Leslee J. Shaw, PhD; Eileen Handberg, PhD; George Sopko, MD; Sheryl F. Kelsey, PhD; Carl J. Pepine, MD; C. Noel Bairey Merz, MD JAMA. 2004;292:1179-1187.

"Cardiorespiratory fitness and adiposity as mortality predictors in older adults." Journal of the American Medical Association, 298(21), 2507-2516. Sui, X., LaMonte, M., Laditka, J., Hardin, J., Chase, N., Hooker, S. & Blair, S. (2007).

"The relationship between low cardiorespiratory fitness and mortality in normal weight, overweight and obese men." JAMA, 282: 1547-1553. Wei, M. Kampert, J.B., Barlow, C.E., et. al (1999).

"Overweight, obesity, mortality in a large prospective cohort of persons 50-71 years old. New England journal of medicine 355 (8), 763-778. Adams, K.F., Schatzkin, A., Harris, t.B., et. al (2006).

"A prospective study of walking as compared to vigorous exercise in the prevention of coronary heart disease." New England Journal of Medicine. 34: 341, 650-658. Manson, J., et. al (1999).

"Brisk Walking and vigorous exercise provide similar cardiovascular disease benefits." European Heart Journal, 21, 1559. Hennekens C.H. (2000).

Chapter Five
"Body image dissatisfaction among third, fourth and fifth grade children." California Journal of Health Promotion, 4 (3), 58-67. Skemp- Artl, K.M. , et. al (2006).

Etiology of body dissatisfaction and weight concerns among 5 year old girls. Apetite, 35 (2), 143-151. Davison, K.K., Markey, C.N. & Birch, L.L. (2000).

"The feeling good handbook." NY: Penguin Putnam books. Burns, D. (1999).

"The 1997 Body Image Survey Results." Psychology Today (30) 30-44. Garner, D (1997, January/February).

Chapter Six
"Teaching Body Confidence." Massachusetts Eating Disorders Association, Boston, MA. Manley, R. (1996).

"Body image dissatisfaction among third, fourth and fifth grade children." California Journal of Health Promotion, 4 (3), 58-67. Skemp- Artl, K.M. , et. al (2006).

"Etiology of body dissatisfaction and weight concerns among 5 year old girls." Apetite, 35 (2), 143-151. Davison, K.K., Markey, C.N. & Birch, L.L. (2000).

Chapter Seven
"Dissociative Symptoms and trauma exposure." Journal of Nervous and Mental Disease, 194, 78-82. Briere, J. (2006).

Chapter Eight
Project EAT 1 and EAT 2 were performed by the Minnesota University School of Public Health. 4700 adolescents and 900 parents were surveyed in 1999. 2,500 of these teens were followed up 5 years later in 2004. Since more than 100 studies were published from this data, we'll send you to their web site rather than cite them all here. The principal researcher was Diane Neumark-Sztainer (2004). (See sph.umn.edu/epi/research/eat/eat-2.asp).

Chapter Nine
"Increased Mortality in Bulimia Nervosa and other Eating Disorders." Am J Psychiatry 2009; 166:1342-1346 Crow, S.J. (2009).

"Latent Structure of eating disorder symptoms: A factor analytic and taxometric investigation." American Journal of Psychiatry, 159, 412-418. Williamson, D.A. et. al (2002).

First and second-order factor structure of the five subscales of the Eating Disorder Inventory. International Journal of Eating Disorders, 23 (2), 189-198. Joiner, T.E. & Heatherton, T.F. (1998).

"Psychiatric comorbidity in patients with eating disorders." Psychological Medicine, 24, 859-867 Braun, D.L., Sunday, S.R. & Halmi, K.A. (1994).

"A longitudinal study of the dietary practices of black and white girls 9 and 10 years old." Journal of Adolescent Health, 27-37. Mellin, L., McNutt, S., Hu, Y., Screiber, G., Crawford, P. & Obarzanek, E. (1991).

"Body image dissatisfaction among third, fourth and fifth grade children." California Journal of Health Promotion, 4 (3), 58-67. Skemp- Artl, K.M. , et. al (2006).

"Etiology of body dissatisfaction and weight concerns among 5 year old girls." Apetite, 35 (2), 143-151. Davison, K.K., Markey, C.N. & Birch, L.L. (2000).

Chapter Ten
"Teaching Body Confidence" Massachusettes Eating disorder Association in Boston, MA. Rebecca Manley (2001).

Epilogue
"Time to value milk." International Journal of Epidemiology, 34 (5). 1160-1162. Elwood, P.C. (2005).

"Benefits of milk powder supplementation of bone accretion in Chinese children." Osteoporosis International, 15 (8), 654-658.
Lau, EMC, Lynn, H, Chan, YH, Lau, W & Woo, J. (2004).

About the Authors

Maria Rago, Ph.D. is a psychologist and the clinical director of Eating Disorders Services at Linden Oaks Hospital at Edwards. She is president of Rago & Associates Counseling Services in Naperville, Illinois, and serves on the Board of Directors of ANAD (Anorexia Nervosa and Associated Disorders). Coca Cola, movie popcorn (with butter, of course), and cheeseburgers rank as her favorite foods.

Greg Archer, OCD, is Editor-in-Chief of the weekly *Good Times Santa Cruz*. His profiles on celebrities, and health and eco patriots – near and far – have appeared in Oprah Magazine, The Advocate, Bust, and The Huffington Post. He also writes about the arts for the *San Francisco Examiner* and moonlights as a certified Spin instructor. Mocha chais, Polish dumplings (with melted butter, of course) and thin-crust Chicago-style pizza make him very happy.

Maria and Greg have been close friends since high school. They lived across the street from each other in Elmhurst, Illinois, but never imagined they would write a book together.

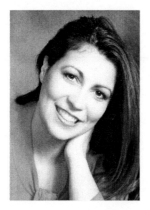 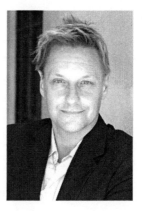

Available from NorlightsPress and fine booksellers everywhere

Toll free: 888-558-4354   **Online:** www.norlightspress.com

Shipping Info: Add $2.95 for first item and $1.00 for each additional item

Name _____

Address _____

Daytime Phone _____

E-mail _____

No. Copies	Title	Price (each)	Total Cost
	Subtotal		
	Shipping		
	Total		

Payment by (circle one):

Check   Visa   Mastercard   Discover   Am Express

Card number_____3 digit code_____

Exp.date_____ Signature_____

Mailing Address:

2721 Tulip Tree Rd.
Nashville, IN 47448

Sign up to receive our catalogue at
www.norlightspress.com

CPSIA information can be obtained at www.ICGtesting.com
Printed in the USA
236016LV00005B/49/P

9 781935 254324